Lokeshwar Chaurasia

Efficacy of Sodium Valproate and Olanzapine in BPD.Mania

Cover image: www.ingimage.com

Publisher:
LAP LAMBERT Academic Publishing
is a trademark of
International Book Market Service Ltd., member of OmniScriptum Publishing Group
17 Meldrum Street, Beau Bassin 71504, Mauritius

Printed at: see last page
ISBN: 978-3-330-32870-9

LIST OF ABBREVIATIONS

BPD	Bipolar Disorder
CBZ	Carbamazepine
COMS-TH	College of Medical Sciences – Teaching Hospital
DSM	Diagnostic and Statistical Manual
DVP	Divalproex
FDA	Food and Drug Administration
GABA	Gamma amino butyric acid
HRSD	Hamilton Rating Scale for Depression
HRQL	Health-related quality of life
ICD	International Classification of Diseases
Li	Lithium
OLZ	Olanzapine
SVA	Sodium valproate
TG1	Treatment group 1
TG2	Treatment group 2
VA	Valproic acid
WHO	World Health Organization
YMRS	Young Mania Rating Scale

LIST OF TABLES

INTRODUCTION

Bipolar disorder (BPD) is a mood disorder that is characterized by periods of pathologic mood elevation (mania or hypomania).[1] The International Classification of Diseases-10 (ICD-10) and Diagnostic and Statistical Manual-IV (DSM-IV) classifications consider mania as a uni-dimensional illness.[2] BPD can be described as a chronic mental illness with marked mood and behavioural dysfunction. The illness is characterised by frequent episodes of relapse and/or recurrence and not much is known about factors that may precipitate new episodes.[3] According to World Health Organization (WHO), BPD is the sixth leading cause worldwide of disability-adjusted life years in individuals aged 15 to 44 years.[4]

The typical period of BPD onset as a syndrome is between 16 and 24 years of age.[5] By the conventional fully-syndromal criteria, the condition becomes less prevalent with increasing age. Bipolar spectrum disorders affect 0.1% of children and 1% of adolescents.[6] The current prototype for this illness is well-characterized for adults and has four cardinal features: (1) episodes of major depression; interspersed to greater or lesser degree with (2) episodes of mania (3) intervals between episodes whose duration, mood state and quality of functioning vary widely between patients and (4) an overall course of psychiatric illness that is chronic.[1,6,7]

Sign and symptoms of mania: a) increased energy, activity and restlessness b) excessively high, overly good, euphoric mood c) extreme irritability d) racing thoughts and talking very fast, jumping from one idea to another e) distractibility, cannot concentrate well f) little sleep needed g) unrealistic beliefs in one's abilities and powers h) poor judgment i) spending sprees j) a lasting period of behavior that is different from usual k) increased sexual drive l) abuse of drugs, particularly cocaine,

1

alcohol and sleeping medications m) provocative, intrusive or aggressive behavior n) denial that anything is wrong.[7]

Although the commonly held opinion is that onset and prevalence of mania decreases with age, there is contradictory evidence that, particularly in men, the incidence of new onset mania increases with age. Clinically, the diagnosis and treatment of geriatric mania is challenging because these patients present with comorbid medical, neurologic and dementing illnesses.[8] Today, two types are officially recognized, BPD type I and type II (BPD-I and BPD-II) and combined they account for a prevalence rate of 3.7% or higher.[9,10]

Many studies have proved that effective pharmacological treatment improves the quality of life in patients suffering with BPD.[11-14] Various classes of antipsychotics and antiepileptics have been used in the treatment of BPD like sodium valproate (SVA), carbamazepine (CBZ), olanzapine (OLZ), risperidone etc.[15,16]

Lithium (Li) was first used to treat manic episodes in the late 1940s, despite Li's marked antimanic activity, response to the drug has been inadequate in almost half of the patients with bipolar illness. The antimanic and antidepressant effects of the anticonvulsants valproate (VLP) and CBZ were found to be therapeutically useful in people with BPDs.[17]

Sodium valproate has mood stabilizing action,[18] whereas olanzapine is an atypical neuroleptic effective in treating both phases of BPD compared with placebo and as effective as established drug therapies.[11] Valproic acid (VA) has actions on gamma amino butyric acid (GABA) and serotonin that link to anti-aggression.[19,20] It is Food and Drug Administration (FDA) approved for the treatment of acute manic episodes

2

and its response rate in acute mania is around 50%, compared to a placebo effect of 20–30%.[21-29] Patients respond relatively rapidly (within 1–2 weeks and often a few days). VLP appears to have a more robust antimanic effect than Li in rapid cycling and mixed episodes.[30,31] Divalproex sodium has been shown to be effective in the treatment of acute manic episodes associated with BPD and is approved by the US FDA for this indication.[25,22] It lacks anticholinergic toxicity, has fewer extra-pyramidal side effects, is associated with a minimal risk of tardive dyskinesia, lacks cardiac and respiratory side effects and has been reported to have better tolerability.[32]

Olanzapine is a derivative and structural analogue of clozapine with a high affinity for dopaminergic (D_1, D_2, D_4), serotonergic, muscarinic, histaminic and α_1 adrenergic receptors.[33] It is antagonistic at both the D_2 and $5\text{-}HT_{2A}$ receptors.[34] It has a solid basis supporting its use in BPD.[35] Some of the side effects of OLZ are weight gain, sedation, orthostatic hypotension and constipation. It is second only to clozapine in causing weight gain.[36]

Despite the introduction of many new mood stabilizing medications and a continually advancing understanding of their individual strengths and weaknesses, selecting the best possible treatment for each individual patient remains a significant challenge for general practitioners and psychiatrists. Response and remission are key goals in the management of BPD, mania.

There are very few literatures related to the direct head to head comparison of SVA and OLZ in bipolar affective disorder, mania and it is a new study in Nepal. Therefore an attempt was made primarily to compare the efficacy of two mood stabilizers- SVA and OLZ using the Young Mania Rating Scale (YMRS) as the scale for assessment.

REVIEW OF LITERATURE

BPD is now recognized as a potentially treatable psychiatric illness with substantial morbidity and mortality and high social and economic impact.[37] Therapies must address the control of acute episodes (manic, depressed or mixed) and maintenance of remission of symptoms. Drug treatments have included Li, anticonvulsants and antipsychotics, but current therapies have proven inadequate for many patients. Only half of bipolar patients achieve remission over two years and half of these relapse within two years.[38]

Historical background

BPD has been known to mankind since the time of the ancient Greeks, but it was not until the 20th century that it was truly recognized as an illness distinct from other psychiatric disorders.

BPD, previously called manic-depressive disorder, is by no means a new illness; it has captured the interest of scholars since the ancient times.[39] It is broadly understood as periods of mania and depression in the same person.[40]

GraecoL Roman Concepts of Mania and Melancholia

The Hippocratic writers understood mania and melancholia as humoral imbalances–melancholia indicating an excess of black bile and mania indicating an excess of yellow bile.[4]

Angst and Marenos identified four distinct meanings of "mania" used during the classical period. [41]

1. A reaction to an event with the meaning of rage, anger or excitation.

4

2. A biologically defined disease.

3. A divine state.

4. A kind of temperament, especially in its mild form.

Healy suggested that, "melancholia was an earlier stage or mild form of madness while mania was the term used for later and more severe stages".[42]

The Nineteenth Century: Falret and Baillarger

In a paper published in 1854 Healy expanded his discussion of "Folie Circulaire"–a circular madness consisting of periods of mania and depression.[42] In the same year Jules Baillarger, proposed a similar category–folie à double forme and demonstrated that there was a single disease and not two; the two supposed attacks were nothing but two stages of a single attack.[42,43]

In 1966, publications supporting the differentiation between unipolar and BPDs brought about the 'rebirth' of BPD.[41] Pichot described 1966 as the year of the "rebirth" of BPD.[40] The third edition of The American Psychiatric Associations Diagnostic and Statistical Manual of Mental Disorders (DSM-III) marked the first formal recognition of BPD as a distinct entity.[44]

Whilst the WHO, 9th edition of the International Classification of Diseases (ICD-9) did not formally incorporate this bipolar –unipolar distinction.[45] The widespread acceptance of BPD as a distinct entity can be seen through its inclusion in ICD-10[2] and its continued place in future editions of Diagnostic and Statistical Manual of Mental Disorders (DSM), including the revised edition of DSM-III (DSM-III-R)[46], as well as DSM-IV[47], DSM-IV-TR[1] and DSM-5.[48]

Bipolar "Disorder" in DSM-IV

BPDs are classified in DSM-IV as mood disorders–"disorders that have a disturbance in mood as the predominant feature".[1] Currently, there are four major subtypes of this disorder in the DSM-IV-Text Revision: bipolar I, bipolar II, cyclothymia and bipolar not otherwise specified.[1]

Bipolar I disorder is characterized by one or more manic or mixed episodes, usually accompanied by major depressive episodes. Bipolar II disorder, by contrast is characterized by one or more major depressive episodes accompanied by at least one hypomanic episode.

Cyclothymic disorder is a chronic, fluctuating mood disturbance involving numerous periods of hypomanic and depressive symptoms.

Bipolar not otherwise specified includes bipolar features that do not meet criteria for any specific BPD.

MANIA

The word derives from the Greek μανία (mania), "madness, frenzy" and that from the verb μαίνομαι (mainomai), "to be mad, to rage, to be furious".[49] Mania is the mood of an abnormally elevated arousal energy level, or "a state of heightened overall activation with enhanced affective expression together with lability of affect".[50]

Elevated irritability is common along with behavior that seems on the surface to be the opposite of depression. Mania is most often associated with BPD, where episodes of mania may alternate unpredictably with episodes of depression or periods of euthymia. It varies in intensity, from mild mania (hypomania) to full mania with extreme energy, racing thoughts and forced speech.[51]

PREVALENCE

Classic prevalence rate was estimated to be 0.8% to 1.7% for full mania and appear comparable across cultures.[10,52] Low lifetime prevalence rates of hypomania have been reported to range between 0.5% and 1.9%.[10] Current literatures suggest that bipolar affects at least 5% of the general population.[53,54]

CLASSIFICATION OF MANIA:

1. Mixed states: In a mixed state the individual has co-occurring manic and depressive features.

2. Hypomania: Is a lowered state of mania that does little to impair function or decrease quality of life.[55]

3. Associated disorders: A single manic episode is sufficient to diagnose bipolar I disorder. Hypomania may be indicative of bipolar II disorder or cyclothymia.

According to ICD-10[2] mania is classified as: F30 Manic episode

F30.0: Hypomania

F30.1: Mania without psychotic symptoms

F30.2: Mania with psychotic symptoms

    .20: With mood-congruent psychotic symptoms

    .21: With mood-incongruent psychotic symptoms

F30.8: Other manic episodes

F30.9: Manic episode, unspecified

Signs and symptoms

The DSM-IV-TR states that the essential feature of bipolar I disorder is a clinical course that is characterized by the occurrence of one or more manic or mixed episodes. A manic episode is defined as a distinct period of at least one week, during which mood is abnormally and persistently elevated, expansive or irritable. This mood disturbance must be accompanied by at least three additional symptoms including inflated self-esteem or grandiosity, decreased need for sleep, pressure of speech, flight of ideas, distractibility, increased involvement in goal-directed activities or psychomotor agitation and excessive involvement in pleasurable activities with a high potential for painful consequences. A mixed episode is defined as a period of one week, during which the criteria are met for both a manic episode and a major depressive episode. Mood disturbances for both a manic and mixed episode must be sufficiently severe to cause marked impairment in occupational or usual social functioning, result in hospitalization or have psychotic features.[1]

The WHO classification system defines a manic episode as one where mood is higher than the person's situation warrants and may vary from relaxed high spirits to barely controllable exuberance, accompanied by hyperactivity, a compulsion to speak, a reduced sleep requirement, difficulty sustaining attention and often increased distractibility. Frequently, confidence and self-esteem are excessively enlarged and grand, extravagant ideas are expressed.[2]

In order to be classified as a manic episode there must be either marked impairment in occupational or social functioning or in the persons relationships with others, an necessitation of hospitalization in order to prevent harm to self or others or psychosis must be present. Psychotic experiences in cases of mania may include grandiose delusions or hallucinations. Such experiences are usually mood congruent– "the content of the delusions or hallucinations is consistent with the manic themes".[1]

Some people also have physical symptoms, such as sweating, pacing and weight loss. In full-blown mania, often the manic person will feel as though his or her goal(s) trump all else, that there are no consequences or that negative consequences would be minimal and that they need not exercise restraint in the pursuit of what they are after.[1]

Hypomania is different, as it may cause little or no impairment in function. The hypomanic person's connection with the external world and its standards of interaction remain intact, although intensity of moods is heightened. But those who suffer from prolonged unresolved hypomania do run the risk of developing full mania and indeed may cross that "line" without even realizing they have done so.[56]

One of the most signature symptoms of mania (and to a lesser extent, hypomania) is what many have described as racing thoughts. These are usually instances in which the manic person is excessively distracted by objectively unimportant stimuli.[57]

Mania is always relative to the normal rate of intensity of the person being diagnosed with it. Other often-less-obvious elements of mania include delusions (of grandeur, potential, persecution, arrogance), hypersensitivity, hypervigilance, hypersexuality, hyper-religiosity, hyperactivity, impulsiveness, compulsion to over explain (keep talking with rapid speech), grandiose ideas and plans and difficulty falling asleep or decreased need for sleep. In manic and hypomanic cases, the afflicted person may engage in out-of-character behavior, which may increase stress in personal relationships, lead to problems at work and increase the risk of altercations with law enforcement. There is a high risk of impulsively taking part in activities potentially harmful to self and others.[58]

Manic patients are frequently grandiose, obsessive, impulsive, irritable, belligerent and frequently deny anything is wrong with them. Because mania frequently encourages high energy and decreased perception of need or ability to sleep, within a few days of a manic cycle, sleep-deprived psychosis may appear, further complicating the ability to think clearly. Racing thoughts and misperceptions lead to frustration and decreased ability to communicate with others.

There are different "stages" or "states" of mania. A minor state is essentially hypomania and like hypomania's characteristics, may involve increased creativity, wit, gregariousness and ambition. Full-blown mania will make a person feel elated, but perhaps also irritable, frustrated and even disconnected from reality.

PATHOPHYSIOLOGY OF MANIA

The biological mechanism by which mania occurs is not yet known. Based on the mechanism of action of antimanic agents (such as antipsychotics, VLP, tamoxifen, Li, CBZ, etc.) and abnormalities seen in patients experiencing a manic episode the following is theorized to be involved in the pathophysiology of mania:

- Dopamine D_2 receptor overactivity (which is a pharmacologic mechanism of antipsychotics in mania).[59]
- Glycogen synthase kinase-3 (GSK-3) overactivity.[60]
- Protein kinase C overactivity. [61]
- Inositol monophosphatase overactivity.[59]
- Increased arachidonic acid turnover. [59]
- Increased cytokine synthesis.[62]

Imaging studies have shown that the left amygdala is more active in women who are manic and the orbitofrontal cortex is less active.[63]

10

SODIUM VALPROATE (SVA)

2.1 Chemical structure

Chemical formula: sodium 2-propylpentanoate

Molecular mass: 166.30 g/mol   Empirical formula: $C_8H_{15}NaO_2$

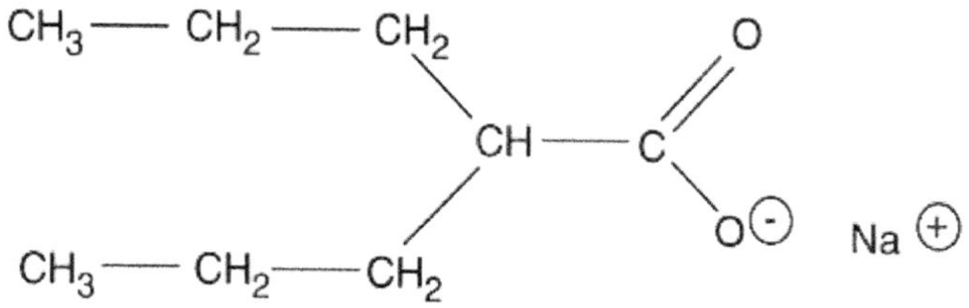

Figure 2.1: Chemical structure of Sodium valproate.

2.2 Chemistry

Sodium valproate or VLP sodium is the sodium salt of valproic acid (VA), also known as valproate or n-dipropylacetic acid or 2-propylpentanoic acid. It is a simple branched-chain carboxylic acid and is also used as the free acid, valproic acid.

It was found to have antiseizure properties when it was used as a solvent in the search for other drugs effective against seizures. It was marketed in France in 1969 but was not licensed in USA until 1978. VA is fully ionized at body pH and for that reason the active form of the drug may be assumed to be the VA ion regardless of whether VA or a salt of the acid is administered.[64]

In 1996, Valproate (VLP) received approval in the United States for use in acute mania. The indications for VLP currently recognized by US FDA are (1) the treatment of the manic episodes associated with BPD, as well as other psychiatric conditions requiring the administration of a mood stabilizer. (2) Sole and adjunctive therapy for

11

complex partial seizures that occur either in isolation or in association with other types of seizures, sole and adjunctive therapy for simple and complex absence seizures and adjunctive therapy for multiple seizure that includes absence seizures and (3) Prophylaxis of migraine headaches.

Four oral preparations of VLP are currently marketed in the United States: VA; sodium syrup; Divalproex (DVP), an enteric-coated stable coordination compound composed of SVA and VA in a 1 to 1 molar relationship and DVP sprinkle capsules, which may be opened and sprinkled on food. An intravenous form (Depacon) is also available for use.

2.3 MECHANISM OF ACTION

The mechanism by which VLP exerts its therapeutic effect is not well understood. Several hypotheses have been proposed concerning the mechanism of action in epilepsy and BPD. The most well studied and understood mechanism of VLP to mediate both its antiepileptic effects and its psychiatric effects, is its ability to potentiate or mimic the effects of inhibitory neurotransmitter, GABA function in central nervous system.[65,66]

GABA is the major inhibitory neurotransmitter in the mammalian central nervous system. VLP inhibits the catabolism of GABA, increases its release, decreases GABA turnover, increases GABA type B (GABA$_B$) receptor density and may also enhance neuronal responsiveness to GABA.[67] Indirectly, this potentiation of GABA has been hypothesized to produce inhibitory effects on central dopamine.[65,66]

Some of the other and less well understood mechanisms involve the inhibition of neuronal excitability and a resultant anti-kindling effect.[65]

One specific area of study has focused on the inhibition of protein kinase C epsilon (PKC-epsilon). PKC-epsilon has been linked to the stimulation of intracellular calcium release and an increase in cortical excitation and instability.[68] VLP has also exhibited effects producing the blockade of voltage-dependent sodium channels.[65,69]

Another proposed mechanism, though controversial, is one likening of VLP to Li as a potential inhibitor of inositol synthesis through inhibition of myoinositol-1phosphate (MIP). It is not well understood if VLP inhibits MIP directly, but it has been shown to deplete inositol.[70,71]

Other effects of VLP that might contribute to its mood-stabilizing properties include decreased dopamine turnover, altered serotonin function, decreased N-methyl-d-aspartate (NMDA) mediated currents, decreased aspartate release and decreased cerebrospinal fluid somatostatin concentrations.[67]

2.4 ABSORPTION, FATE AND EXCRETION

SVA is well absorbed following an oral dose from gastrointestinal tract with bioavailability greater than 80%. Its rate of absorption may vary with the formulation administered, conditions of use and the method of administration. Peak blood levels are observed within 2 hours.

It is 90% bound to plasma proteins, although the fraction bound is somewhat reduced at blood levels greater than 150 mcg/mL. Since SVA is both highly ionized and highly protein-bound, its distribution is essentially confined to extracellular water with a volume of distribution of approximately 0.15 L/kg. Higher than expected free fractions occur in elderly, in hyperlipidemic patients and in patients with hepatic and renal diseases.

Clearance for SVA is low, its half-life varies from 9 hours to 18 hours. SVA is metabolized almost entirely by the liver. In adult patients on monotherapy, 30-50% of an administered dose appears in urine as a glucuronide conjugate. Mitochondrial ß-oxidation is the other major metabolic pathway, typically accounting for over 40% of the dose. Usually, less than 15-20% of the dose is eliminated by other oxidative mechanisms. Less than 3% of an administered dose is excreted unchanged in urine.[67]

2.5 DOSAGE AND ADMINISTRATION

In acutely manic adolescents and adults, SVA treatment may be begun via the oral-loading strategy of 20 to 30 mg/kg a day so that therapeutic concentrations can be achieved on the first day of treatment, often with rapid onset of response and minimal adverse effects. However, in patients who are euthymic, hypomanic, depressed, very young or elderly, VLP treatment should be initiated in lower, divided doses (e.g. 250 to 750 mg a day in adolescents and adults and 125 to 250 mg a day in children and elderly adults) to minimize gastrointestinal and neurological toxicity. Patients who cannot swallow pills, particularly children and elderly adults, can use DVP sprinkle capsules. The VLP dose is then titrated upward according to response and adverse effects, generally to a serum concentration between 50 to 150 µg/mL. Once patients are stabilized, VLP dosage regimens can often be simplified to once daily dose, usually taken at night, to enhance convenience and compliance.[67]

2.6 ADVERSE EFFECTS

Minor adverse effects

The most frequent side effects at the beginning of treatment with SVA are gastrointestinal (nausea, dyspepsia, vomiting, and diarrhea) and neurological (sedation, ataxia, dysarthria and tremor) which often decrease with time. It frequently produces modest elevations in hepatic transaminases. Other bothersome side effects are weight gain and hair loss.

Serious adverse effects

In very rare cases, causes fatal hepatotoxicity, hemorrhagic pancreatitis, agranulocytosis, encephalopathy with coma and skeletal muscle weakness with respiratory failure. It may cause coma and death when taken in overdose.

2.7 TOXICITY

For oral route in mouse, the $LD_{50} = 1098$ mg/kg and in rat, the $LD_{50} = 670$ mg/kg. The safety and tolerability of VLP in pediatric patients were shown to be comparable to those in adults.

2.8 DRUG INTERACTION

2.8.1 SVA with other drugs

SVA tends to inhibit the clearance of other concomitant drugs metabolized in the liver. Conversely, it may increase the concentration of phenobarbital and probably other barbiturates by impairing non-renal clearance.

Because it is highly protein bound, serum VLP free fraction concentrations can be increased and it's toxicity be precipitated by co-administration of other highly protein-bound drugs (e.g., aspirin, CBZ, diazepam) that can displace VLP from its protein-binding sites.

Since VLP inhibits the secondary phase of platelet aggregation, it should be used cautiously in combination with other drugs that affect coagulation, such as warfarin and aspirin.

2.8.2 SVA and other psychotropic drugs

In general, combinations of SVA with Li, antipsychotics, antidepressants, CBZ, gabapentin, lamotrigine, topiramate and benzodiazepines are well tolerated and often appear to be more effective than SVA used alone. The combination of SVA and typical antipsychotics is also commonly used, especially in acutely manic patients. Although SVA and antipsychotics do not appear to affect the plasma concentrations of one another significantly, the combination may evoke increased sedation and increase antipsychotic-induced extrapyramidal effects which may be treated by antipsychotic dosage reduction or by the addition of an antiparkinsonian agent.

Clozapine may also be combined with VLP which is well tolerated, with sedation being the most frequent adverse reaction. Increasing clinical experience suggests that VLP may also be safely combined with other atypical antipsychotics, including OLZ, risperidone, quetiapine and sertindole.[67]

Antidepressants including tricyclic drugs, monoamine oxidase inhibitors, selective serotonin reuptake inhibitors and other agents are frequently combined with VLP, usually without difficulty. However, the tricyclic amitriptyline increases VLP serum concentrations, possibly by increasing the binding of VLP to tissue. Conversely, VLP increases the levels of tricyclic drugs, presumably by inhibiting their metabolism.

When combined with benzodiazepines or CBZ, VLP may compete for protein-binding sites, serum concentrations of unbound diazepam and CBZ increases. However, lorazepam is apparently not displaced in that manner. The combination of VLP and clonazepam has been reported to produce absence status.

OLANZAPINE

2.9 CHEMICAL STRUCTURE

Chemical formula:

2-methyl-4-(4-methyl-1-piperazinyl)-10H-thieno [2, 3-b][1,5] benzodiazepine

Molecular mass: 312.439 g/mol   Empirical formula: $C_{17}H_{20}N_4S$

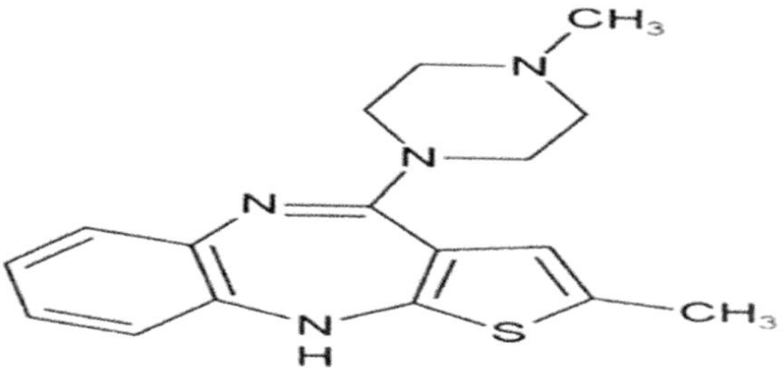

Figure 2.2: Chemical structure of Olanzapine.

2.10 Chemistry

It is a thieno-benzodiazepine analog and is an achiral substance, present as yellow, crystalline powder. It is practically insoluble in water and soluble in dichloromethane, chloroform, acetone, dimethylsulfoxide, dimethylacetamide, N-methyl pyrrolidone and in water at pH < 2.

OLZ is an atypical antipsychotic, approved by the United States FDA for the treatment of schizophrenia and BPD in October 1996.[72] It is recommended by the National Institute of Health and Care Excellence as a first line therapy for the treatment of acute mania in BPD. Other recommended first lines are haloperidol, quetiapine and risperidone.[73] The Network for Mood and Anxiety

17

Treatments (CANMAT) recommends OLZ as a first line maintenance treatment in BPD.[74] It is effective in treating the acute exacerbations of schizophrenia.[75]

It is no less effective than Li or VLP and is more effective than placebo in treating BPD.[76]

2.11 MECHANISM OF ACTION

OLZ is an atypical antipsychotic, antimanic and mood stabilizing agent that demonstrates a broad pharmacological profile across a number of receptor systems. It displays a very broad pharmacological profile with potent activity and wide range of receptor affinities for serotonin $5HT_{2A/2C}$, $5HT_3$, $5HT_6$; dopamine D_1, D_2, D_3, D_4, D_5; cholinergic muscarinic receptors M_1-M_5; α_1 adrenergic and histamine H_1 receptors.[77,78,79,80,81] Its antagonism to muscarinic receptors may explain its anticholinergic properties.

Animal behavioral studies show that OLZ has atypical antipsychotic characteristics, by virtue of its in vitro receptor profile.[77,78,79,80,81] The drug demonstrated a greater in vitro affinity for serotonin $5HT_2$ than dopamine D_2 receptors and in in vivo models, greater $5HT_2$ affinity than D_2 activity.

In addition OLZ also binds to GABA α_1 receptor and the benzodiazepine binding sites.[34]

OLZ's antipsychotic and mood-stabilizing effects are likely the result of potent antagonism at dopamine and serotonin receptors with affinity constants ranging from 4 nM to 31 nM. It also binds with high affinity to H_1 and M_1 receptors. It binds with moderate affinity to $5-HT_3$ and M_{2-5} receptors and binds weakly to GABA, benzodiazepine binding sites and β-adrenergic receptors. It is also likely that the drug

18

regulates various signaling pathways within the brain, including the extracellular signal-related kinases (ERK 1/2) particularly with long-term treatment.[82]

2.12 ABSORPTION, FATE AND EXCRETION

OLZ is well absorbed after oral administration from gastrointestinal tract with bioavailability of 87% and reaches peak blood levels in about 5 hours in adults. Eating does not appear to affect its bioavailability.[83]

It is highly protein bound (about 93%) with a volume of distribution of 10-18 L/kg. About 40% is metabolized in the liver through first pass, to inactive metabolites mainly by cytochrome P450 isozyme CYP1A2, flavin-containing monooxygenase (FMO) 3 and N-glucuronidation. Minor pathways involve CYP2D6 and possibly CYPS2C19 isozymes. Because of the number of possible routes of metabolism, inhibition of cytochrome oxidase pathways does not markedly affect its elimination. Within the liver, it undergoes glucuronidation, allylic hydroxylation, oxidation and dealkylation. The major metabolites found in humans are 10-N-glucuronide and 4-desmethylolanzapine.[84]

Plasma levels of OLZ appear to increase slowly over a period of months with a slightly slower time course in women compared with men. The elimination half-life ranges from about 27 hours in smokers to 37 hours in nonsmokers.[85] The concentration-to-dose ratio of OLZ appears generally linear.[84] However, adolescents appear to have a higher (~34%) concentration-to-dose ratio than adults even after adjustment for weight.[85]

It is excreted in the urine (65%) and feces (35%) over the course of ~7 days.[83]

2.13 DOSAGE AND ADMINISTRATION

OLZ is marketed in a number of countries, with tablets ranging from 2.5 to 20 milligrams. It is marketed as a tablet with trade names like Lanzek, Oleanz, Zyprexa etc. Its antipsychotic efficacy is demonstrated in the dose range of 5-20 mg/day.

- It can be taken once a day in doses of 2.5 mg, 5 mg, 7.5 mg, 10 mg, 15 mg and 20 mg. It is well tolerated by most people and can be taken with or without meals. No routine blood level monitoring is required.

- OLZ orally disintegrating tablets that dissolves in the mouth on contact with saliva, is available as 5mg, 10mg, 15mg and 20mg tablets. Tablets can be taken with or without water.

- Short-term treatment with intramuscular OLZ is used to treat agitation (overexcited, hostile or threatening behavior) in people with schizophrenia or BPD.

Usual monotherapy dose of oral OLZ should be administered on a once-a-day schedule without regard to meals, generally beginning with 10 or 15 mg. Dosage adjustments, if indicated, should generally occur at intervals of not less than 24 hours. When dosage adjustment is necessary, dose increments/decrements of 5 mg on prescription is recommended.

2.14 Adverse effects

The principal side effect of OLZ is weight gain, which may be profound in some cases and/or associated with derangement in the blood lipid and blood sugar profiles. The weight gain has been linked to genetic variations in the 5-HT$_{2A}$, 5-HT$_{2C}$, β_3-adrenergic receptor, leptin and the G-protein β_3 subunit genes.[86,87] It's metabolic adverse effects have been hypothesized to be related to its histaminergic binding profile.[88]

System wise adverse effects of OLZ include:

Cardiovascular system: postural hypotension, tachycardia, chest pain, hypotension.

Central nervous system: somnolence, agitation, insomnia, headache, nervousness, hostility, dizziness, anxiety, personality disorder, akathisia, hypertonia, speech disorder, tremor, amnesia, drug dependence, euphoria, neurosis, seizures, aggression.

Endocrine system: weight gain, increased appetite, fever, edema, peripheral edema, transient prolactin elevation, menstrual disorder, hyperglycemia, diabetes mellitus, neuroleptic malignant syndrome. Uric acid may also increase.

Gastrointestinal system: abdominal pain, constipation, dry mouth.

Hematologic: Leukopenia, neutropenia, transient eosinophilia, agranulocytosis and pancytopenia.

Hepatic: Increased levels of Alanine transaminase (ALT), Aspartate anino transferase (AST), Gamma glutamyl transpeptidase(GGT).

Neuromuscular: arthralgia, joint disorders, twitching, neck rigidity, back pain, increased creatine kinase.

Other adverse effects: rhinitis, increased cough, pharyngitis, amblyopia, blepharitis, corneal lesions, pancreatitis, vesiculobullous rash, dermatitis, priapism.

Extrapyramidal side effects: although potentially serious are infrequent to rare, but may include tardive dyskinesia, tremors and muscle rigidity.[89] It may produce non-trivial hyperglycemia in patients with diabetes mellitus. Likewise, the elderly are at a greater risk of falls and accidental injury. Young males appear to be at heightened risk of dystonic reactions.

2.15 Toxicity

Symptoms of an overdose include tachycardia, agitation, dysarthria, decreased consciousness and coma. Death has been reported after an acute overdose of 450 mg, but also survival after an acute overdose of 2000 mg has been found.[90]

2.16 Drug interactions

Diazepam when co-administered with OLZ potentiates orthostatic hypotension. Increased clearance of OLZ occurs with CBZ therapy, fluoxetine, rifampin and omeprazole whereas it decreases with fluvoxamine.

The pharmacokinetic parameters of OLZ are not affected by warfarin, Li, VLP, alcohol, imipramine, biperidin, theophylline so dosing adjustments is not required. Its bioavailability is not affected by cimetidine and antacids.

OLZ enhances the actions of antihypertensive agents and also produces somnolence when co-administered with lorazepam. It antagonizes levodopa and dopamine agonists.

Its plasma level is affected by smoking (leading to ~30% reduction in plasma level), gender (women have ~85% increased plasma levels), CBZ (decreased plasma levels), fluvoxamine and other selective serotonin reuptake inhibitors (increased plasma levels).[91,92,93]

Most controlled clinical trials of pharmacological treatment for bipolar affective disorder, mania focus on short-term improvement, collecting data for only 3–6 weeks. Examining data from only the first few weeks of medication use may lead to incorrectly concluding that medications with more rapid onset of action are more efficacious than those with slower onset.[94]

Drug treatments have included Li, anticonvulsants and antipsychotics, but current therapies have proven inadequate for many patients, only half of bipolar patients achieve remission over two years and half of these relapse within the two years.[38]

Tariot et al.[95] conducted a 6-week, multicenter, randomized, double-blind, placebo-controlled, parallel-group study to assess the efficacy, tolerability and safety of DVP sodium in the treatment of elderly patients with dementia who exhibited manic symptoms. The study concluded that DVP sodium did not improve signs and symptoms of mania associated with dementia in this sample of nursing-home residents, but did improve symptoms of agitation.

Pope et al.[25] conducted a placebo-controlled, double-blind study on VLP in the treatment of acute mania. Patients (n=17) randomized to active drug demonstrated a median 54% decrease in scores on the YMRS as compared with a median 5.0% decrease among the patients (n=19) receiving placebo. The study showed that VLP proved superior to placebo in alleviating manic symptoms and concluded that VLP represents a useful new drug for the treatment of manic patients.

Hirscfeld et al.[9] conducted a pooled analysis, from 3 randomized, double-blind, parallel-group, active- or placebo-controlled studies to compare the efficacy, safety and tolerability of oral-loaded DVP with standard-titration DVP, Li, OLZ or placebo. The analysis concluded that the oral loading of DVP leads to a more rapid antimanic effect when compared with standard-titration DVP, Li or placebo and is better tolerated than OLZ and as well tolerated as Li or standard-titration DVP.

Ozcan et al.[96] conducted an open label, clinical comparative study with inpatients to test whether the clinical effectiveness and the time for onset of action of Li, CBZ and VLP in acute mania is different or not. All of study drugs reduced assessment scale scores significantly at the end of third week. The study concluded that Li, CBZ and VLP are efficacious antimanic agents that have no superiority on each other in treatment of acute mania.

Müller-Oerlinghausen et al.[97] conducted a prospective, randomized, double-blind, placebo-controlled, multicenter study to compare the efficacy of SVA administered as adjunct to neuroleptic medication for patients with acute mania with the efficacy of neuroleptics alone. The study concluded that the combination of neuroleptic and VLP was superior to neuroleptics in attempts to alleviate manic symptoms. VLP represents a useful adjunct medication for the treatment of acute manic symptoms (50% improvement rate on the YMRS).

A study conducted by Kusumakar et al.[98] to summarize the quality of evidence for the efficacy of different biological treatments in mania, mixed state and rapid cycling and to propose guidelines for treatment of these conditions. The study concluded that Li and DVP sodium were effective in classical pure mania, whereas DVP sodium and CBZ were likely more effective in mixed states. DVP sodium was likely more efficacious than CBZ and Li when the mania was a part of rapid-cycling course.

Xue et al.[99] conducted a systematic literature review on OLZ in Chinese patients with schizophrenia or BPD to examine evidence of the efficacy, effectiveness and safety of OLZ in Chinese populations. The efficacy of OLZ in Chinese populations was confirmed by multiple comparative and non-comparative studies that found statistically significant reductions in symptom measures in studies conducted for ≥ 6 weeks (schizophrenia) or ≥ 3 weeks (BPD). The study concluded that Chinese and non-Chinese populations with schizophrenia or BPD treated with OLZ displayed broadly similar responses.

Poo et al.[100] reviewed the efficacy and tolerability profiles of atypical antipsychotics used to treat adult BPD in clinical practice, in relation to the latest National Institute for Health and Care Excellence guidelines (CG185). The study concluded that OLZ monotherapy and in combination with fluoxetine, quetiapine, risperidone, aripiprazole and asenapine was useful in the management of adult BPD in the subsets of mania, depression or mixed episodes and all of these drugs had anti-manic effects.

Cazorla et al.[101] conducted an exploratory post hoc, pooled analysis to evaluate the potential differential effects over time of asenapine and OLZ compared with placebo on the YMRS, over 21 days in patients with manic or mixed episodes in bipolar I disorder. The study showed each of the eleven individual YMRS item scores was significantly reduced compared with placebo at day 21. After 2 days of treatment, asenapine and OLZ were superior to placebo for six of the YMRS items: disruptive/aggressive behaviour, content, irritability, elevated mood, sleep and speech.

A multicenter, double-blind, randomized, controlled trial conducted by Niufan et al.[102] to examine the efficacy and safety of OLZ versus Li in the treatment of patients with bipolar manic/mixed episodes. Patients with bipolar manic or mixed episode (DSM-IV criteria) and YMRS score ≥ 20 at screening received OLZ (5–20 mg/day, n= 69) or Li carbonate (600–1800 mg/day, n= 71) for 4 weeks. The improvement in symptoms of bipolar mania and rate of response was significantly greater in the OLZ treatment group compared to the Li group, although there was no difference between the two treatment groups in terms of remission rate.

Narasimhan et al.[12] review on OLZ in the management of BPD in which acute mania trials have demonstrated superior efficacy of OLZ to placebo, equal or superior efficacy to VLP and superior efficacy in combination therapy with Li or VLP compared to mood stabilizer monotherapy. The review showed OLZ to be more efficacious than placebo in the prevention of manic and depressive relapses and was non-inferior to Li or VLP; and suggested OLZ as an invaluable addition to the pharmacological armamentarium in the treatment of bipolar I disorder.

Baker et al.[103] conducted a secondary analysis of a 6-week, double-blind, randomised study to evaluate the efficacy of OLZ in combination with Li or VLP, for treating depressive symptoms associated with mania. Total YMRS improvement was superior with OLZ co-therapy. The study concluded that in patients with acute dysphoric mania addition of OLZ to ongoing Li or VLP monotherapy significantly improved depressive symptom, mania and suicidality ratings.

Kumar et al.[15] conducted a study to compare the efficacy of SVA and OLZ administered alone or in combination in patients suffering from acute mania. Patients (n=30) suffering from acute mania were divided into two equal groups. In both groups SVA or OLZ was given as add-on therapy at 3 weeks. SVA and OLZ were effective in the treatment of acute mania, with all patients demonstrating a 50% or more improvement on the YMRS. The study supported combination therapy in the management of acute mania and suggested that serum VA levels of 100 microg/mL was necessary for clinical response.

Tohen et al.[104] conducted a 47-week, randomized, double-blind study comparing flexibly dosed OLZ (5–20 mg/day) to DVP (500–2500 mg/day) for manic or mixed episodes of BPD. The primary efficacy instrument was the YMRS with prioriprotocol-defined threshold scores of ≥20 for inclusion, ≤12 for remission and ≥15 for relapse. There were no significant differences between treatments in the rates of symptomatic mania remission over the 47 weeks (56.8% and 45.5%, respectively) and subsequent relapse into mania or depression (42.3% and 56.5%). The study concluded that symptomatic remission occurred sooner and overall mania improvement was greater for OLZ than for DVP but rates of bipolar relapse did not differ.

A 12-week, double-blind, double-dummy, randomized clinical trial conducted by Reviki et al.[105] to compare the clinical, health-related quality of life (HRQL) and economic outcomes of DVP and OLZ in the treatment of acute mania associated with BPD. The study concluded that DVP was associated with lower 12-week outpatient costs compared with OLZ. DVP and OLZ had similar short-term effects on clinical or HRQL outcomes in BPD subjects.

Tohen et al.[27] conducted a 3-week, randomized, double-blind clinical trial to compare the effects of OLZ and DVP for the treatment of mania, using YMRS and HRSD to quantify manic and depressive symptoms, respectively. The study concluded that OLZ treatment group had significantly greater mean improvement of mania ratings and a significantly greater proportion of patients achieved protocol-defined remission compared with the DVP treatment group.

Zajeka et al.[106] conducted a randomized, 12-week, double-blind, parallel-group, multicenter study which included DSM-IV defined BPD type I patients hospitalized for acute mania and randomly assigned to treatment with DVP or OLZ. MRS was used as assessment scale. The study concluded that there was no significant difference in efficacy between treatment groups. Also DVP was associated with a more favorable adverse event profile and significantly less weight gain than OLZ.

Tohen et al.[107] conducted a double-masked trial for 18 months in patients achieving syndromic remission after 6 week's treatment with OLZ plus either Li (0.6-1.2 mmol/l) or VLP (50-125 mg/ml)received Li or VLP plus either OLZ 5-20 mg/day (combination therapy) or placebo (monotherapy). The study concluded that patients taking OLZ added to Li or VLP experienced sustained symptomatic remission, but not syndromic remission for longer than those receiving Li or VLP monotherapy.

Tohen et al.[108] conducted a 6-week double-blind, randomized, placebo-controlled trial to determine the efficacy of combined therapy with OLZ and either VLP or Li compared with VLP or Li alone in treating acute manic or mixed bipolar episodes. The study concluded that compared with the use of VLP or Li alone, the addition of OLZ provided superior efficacy in the treatment of manic and mixed bipolar episodes.

Cipriani et al.[109] conducted a multiple treatments meta-analysis to assess the effects of all antimanic drugs. 68 randomised controlled trials (16,073 participants) were systematically reviewed. Risperidone and OLZ had a very similar profile of comparative efficacy, being more effective than VLP, ziprasidone, lamotrigine, topiramate and gabapentin. Overall, antipsychotic drugs were significantly more effective than mood stabilizers.

Bai et al.[110] study on Taiwan consensus of pharmacological treatment for BPD showed that, for the acute manic phase 75% of the experts would like to use combination therapy with mood stabilizers (VA or Li) and atypical antipsychotics (quetiapine, risperidone or OLZ). Another 25% of the experts were inclined to use monotherapy with the first choice of DVP, followed by Li and then atypical antipsychotics in the sequence of quetiapine, risperidone and finally OLZ.

Osso et al.[111] conducted a naturalistic study to assess clinical features and long-term response to mood stabilizers in a sample of bipolar subjects with different ages at onset. Mood stabilizer treatment included the following psychotropic compounds: Li, anticonvulsants (i.e VLP and CBZ) and atypical antipsychotics (i.e quetiapine, OLZ and risperidone). The study suggested clinical peculiarities and different patterns of response to mood stabilizers across distinct subgroups of patients with BPD and different ages at onset.

Kim et al.[112] conducted a naturalistic observational study of psychiatric inpatients on weight change in the acute treatment of bipolar I disorder. The study concluded that even during short period of acute treatment, bipolar patients showed significant weight gain and became obese in a closed-ward setting in patients on any kind of atypical antipsychotics than those on typical antipsychotics or without antipsychotics.

Luca et al.[113] conducted a study to evaluate the prevalence of major depression, BPD type I, cyclothymia and dysthymia mood disorders and gender distribution and to relate familiality, comorbidity and marital status to each diagnosis. The study concluded that prescribing patterns for antidepressants, antipsychotics and mood stabilizers in the treatment of mood disorders showed a shift from older to newer drugs and wider use of mood stabilizers.

AIM AND OBJECTIVE OF THE STUDY

To study the efficacy of sodium valproate in comparison to olanzapine in bipolar affective disorder, mania patients in CMS-TH, Bharatpur.

4. METHODOLOGY

4.1 TRIAL DESIGN, PARTICIPANTS AND SAMPLE SIZE

The study was conducted in collaboration with Department of Psychiatry, College of Medical Sciences – Teaching Hospital (CMS-TH), Bharatpur-10, Chitwan during the period of August 2013 to January 2015. The study was done in patients visiting Department of Psychiatry, CMS-TH diagnosed with bipolar affective disorder, mania.

This was a hospital based prospective randomized clinical trial, with two treatment group design.

Ethical clearance was taken from Institutional Review Committee (IRC) of CMS-TH and Kathmandu University.

Out of 74 patients attending the Department of Psychiatry with bipolar affective disorder, mania; 60 patients were included for the study after exclusion and lost follow-up. All the participants were provided with verbal information regarding study protocol and consent form was signed to participate in the study.

Selection was done on the basis of fulfillment of the inclusion and exclusion criteria.

Inclusion criteria:

1. Patients between the ages of 18 and 75 years.

2. All patients diagnosed with clinical bipolar affective disorder mania, DSM-IV-TR Patient Version.

3. Patient's with a minimum total score of 20 on the YMRS,[114] at both the screening visit and on the day of random assignment to study groups (baseline).

4. Patients who provided written consent.

Exclusion criteria:

1.   Patients falling in the age category < 18 years and > 75 years.

2.   Patient with an YMRS score of < 20.

3.   Pregnant and nursing women.

4.   Patients with history of uncontrolled gastrointestinal, renal, hepatic, endocrine, cardiovascular, pulmonary, immunologic or hematologic disease.

5.   Patients with serious or unstable medical illness.

6.   Patients with a history of severe drug allergy or hypersensitivity reactions to the study drugs.

7.   Patients at imminent risk of causing injury to themselves or others.

8.   DSM-IV substance dependence within the past 30 days (except nicotine or caffeine)

All the patients diagnosed with bipolar affective disorder, mania were randomly divided into two treatment groups: Treatment Group 1 (TG1) and Treatment Group 2 (TG2). Sampling technique was simple random sampling. Sample size was measured as 30 patients in each group. TG1 group included the patients receiving SVA (500 to 2500 mg per day) and TG2 group included the patients receiving OLZ (5 to 20 mg per day). The doses of both the drugs to individual patient, assigned by the consulting Psychiatrist were based on sign and symptoms, clinical response, drug plasma levels and adverse events. Patients were informed about the possible side effects of drug. Sample was selected by lottery method with piece of paper marked with 'S' for SVA group and 'O' for OLZ group which were mixed together. These papers were used to randomly allocate the patient in 2 treatment groups at day 0 (baseline).

In the present study, out of 74 patients diagnosed with bipolar affective disorder, mania, a total of 60 patients were studied after exclusion and lost to follow up.

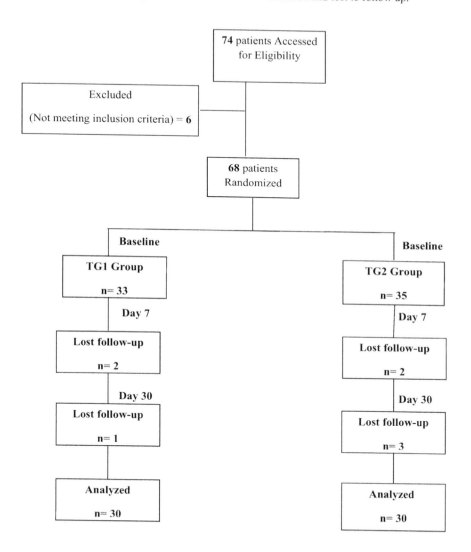

Figure 4.1: Flow diagram of Study design

4.2 ASSESSMENT OF SUBJECTS

Severity of illness was assessed with the 11-item, Young Mania Rating Scale (YMRS).[114] YMRS total score $\leq$ 12 indicates remission of symptoms and clinical response, defined as $\geq$ 50% baseline-to-endpoint reduction in YMRS total score. The most widely used clinician administered rating scale for mania is YMRS. It contains 11 items, four of which are scored 0-4 and the remaining seven are scored from 0-8, based on severity. The YMRS is designed as a 15 to 30 minute's interview administered by trained clinicians. It has been used extensively to assess treatment response in clinical trial studies. It is considered to be the gold standard to which scale developers evaluate concurrent validity with newer scales. The authors report good inter-rater reliability for items ($r = 0.66 - 0.92$) and total scores ($r = 0.93$) and good concurrent validity ($r = 0.71$) with the Mental Status Reporting Software (MSRS)[115] and global ratings ($r = 0.88$). Limitations include the fact that there is no guideline to ensure standardized administration, no report of discriminant validity or test-retest reliability. One criticism raised by Altman is that the YMRS combines symptoms of mania with psychotic symptoms to yield a total score; he suggests that this was troublesome as these symptoms may respond differently to treatment. [116]

Periodic psychiatric assessment was done at every visit. At each visit YMRS was applied to each patient and severity of disease was evaluated on each visit i.e. day 0 (baseline), day 7 and day 30 and was compared to day 0 (baselilne).

4.3 STATISTICAL ANALYSIS

The data was entered in Microsoft Excel Program (Microsoft Office 2007). Statistical analysis was done by SPSS 20.0 version (Statistical Package for Social Science for Windows Version). Descriptive statistical analysis was done in the present study. Results on continuous measurement were presented as Mean ± SD and results on categorical measurement were presented in number and percentage (%). To find the significance of study parameters for single group, Paired Samples t-test was used. Comparison was done at 95% confidence interval of the distribution of the data and p value < 0.05 was considered statistically significant.

OBSERVATION AND RESULTS

DEMOGRAPHIC FEATURES OF STUDY POPULATION

This study enrolled, a total of 60 patients diagnosed with bipolar affective disorder, mania by DSM-IV TR and ICD-10 criteria with 100% completing minimum 30 days duration of therapy, attending Department of Psychiatry at College of Medical Sciences Teaching Hospital (CMS-TH), Bharatpur, Nepal from August 2013 to January 2015.

5.1 AGE AND GENDER

The mean age of male participants was 39.80 ± 15.85 years and the mean age of female participants was 35.14 ± 9.40 years, while the mean age of the study population was 37.08 ± 12.59 years which is depicted by table 5.1 and figure 5.1.

Table 5.1: Mean age of study population

Sex	N	Minimum	Maximum	Mean	Std. Deviation
Male	25	18	70	39.80	15.85
Female	35	20	62	35.14	9.40
Overall		18	70	37.08	12.59

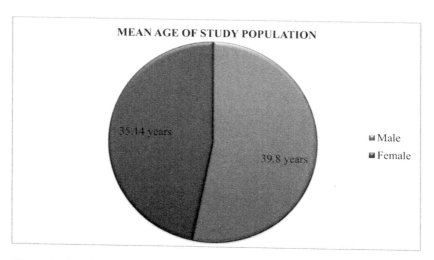

MEAN AGE OF STUDY POPULATION

35.14 years

39.8 years

■ Male
■ Female

Figure 5.1: Pie chart showing mean age of study population.

Table 5.2: Mean age of patient in both the treatment groups

Treatment group	Mean age (in years)	Standard deviation
TG1	36.77	14.258
TG2	37.40	10.912

Statistically no significant difference, p= 0.312

Mean age of the patients in the TG1 was 36.77 ± 14.258 and in TG2 the mean age was 37.40 ± 10.912.

AGE GROUP

In this study, maximum number of patients were in the age group of 28-37 years (35%), com0prising of 14 females and 7 males. Minimum number of patients were found in age group of ≥ 68 years which is depicted in table 5.3 and figure 5.2.

Table 5.3: Age group distribution of study population

Age group (in years)	Frequency (n)	Percentage (%)
18 – 27	14	23.33
28 – 37	21	35.00
38 – 47	14	23.33
48 – 57	6	10.00
58 – 67	4	6.67
≥ 68	1	1.67
Total	60	100

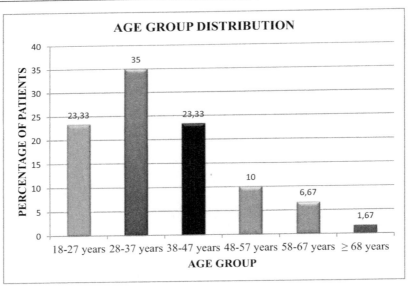

Figure 5.2: Bar diagram showing the age distribution of study population.

Table 5.4: Age wise distribution of study population in different treatment groups

Age Group (in years)	Number of patients in Treatment Group 1 (TG1)	Number of patients in Treatment Group 2 (TG2)
18 – 27	8	6
28 – 37	1	10
38 – 47	6	8
48 – 57	1	5
58 – 67	3	1
≥ 68	1	0
Total	30	30

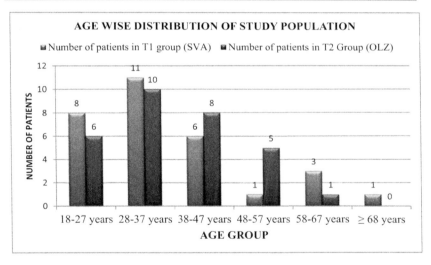

Figure 5.3: Bar Diagram showing the age distribution in both treatment groups.

Maximum number of patients who were treated with SVA belonged to 18-27 years (26.66%) age group and the maximum number of patients who were treated with OLZ belonged to 28-37 years (33.33%) age group.

39

GENDER

Females were the predominant sex 58.3% (n=35) followed by males 41.7% (n=25) of the total study population, showing overall female predominance. Also there was predominance of females in individual treatment groups.

Table 5.5: Gender distribution of study population

Gender	Frequency (n)	Percentage (%)	Number of patients in TG1 (SVA)	Number of patients in TG2 (OLZ)
Male	25	41.7	13	12
Female	35	58.3	17	18
Total	60	100.0	30	30

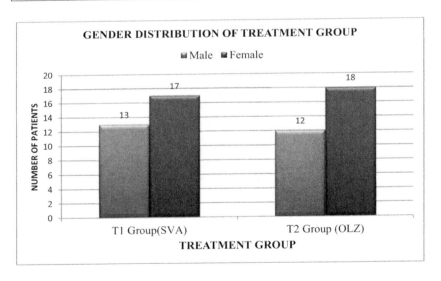

Figure 5.4: Bar diagram showing gender distribution of study population in both the treatment groups.

MARITAL STATUS

Table 5.6: Marital status of study population

Marital status	Frequency (n)	Percentage (%)
Married	41	68.33
Unmarried	19	31.66

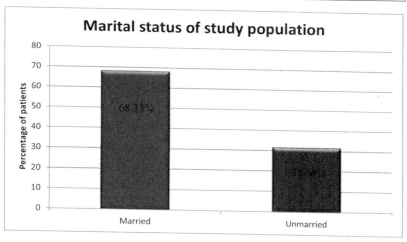

Figure 5.5: Bar diagram showing marital status of study population.

Most of the enrolled patients were married (68.33%) while only 31.66% were unmarried.

RELIGION

Table 5.7: Distribution of study population by religion

Religion	Frequency (n)	Percentage (%)
Hindu	34	56.66
Others	26	43.33

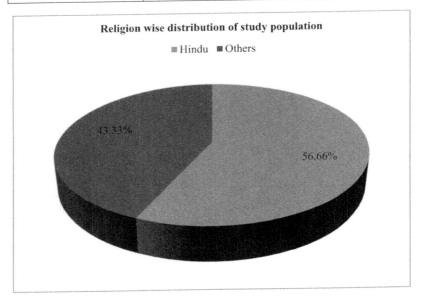

Figure 5.6: Pie chart showing religion wise distribution of study population.

There were 34 hindus who constituted 56.66% and 26 (43.33%) were from other religions.

OCCUPATION

Table 5.8: Occupation distribution of study population

Occupation	Frequency (n)	Percentage (%)
Housewife	21	35
Farmer	16	26.66
Unemployed	10	16.66
Business	7	11.66
Student	6	10

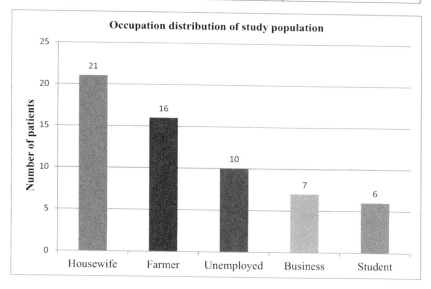

Figure 5.7: Bar diagram showing occupation of study population.

Out of 60 patients involved in the study, 21(35%) were housewives, 16(26.66%) were farmers, 10(16.66%) were unemployed, 7(11.66%) were businessman and 6(10%) were student as shown in table 5.8 and figure 5.7.

SOCIOECONOMIC STATUS: 48.33% of the study population belonged to low SES, 36.66% belonged to middle SES and 15% belonged to low SES as shown in table 5.9 and figure 5.8.

Table 5.9: Socioeconomic status of study population

SES	Frequency (n)	Percentage (%)
Low	29	48.33
Middle	22	36.66
High	9	15

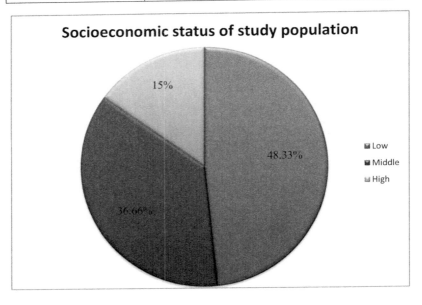

Figure 5.8: Pie chart showing the socioeconomic status of study population.

STARTING DOSES OF SVA

In the present study, 30 bipolar affective disorder, mania patients having different scores on the YMRS, were treated with different doses of SVA ranging from 1000 mg/day to 2000 mg/day. Among them 60% (n=18) were started with 1500 mg/day, 36.66% (n=11) were started with 1000 mg/day and 3.33% (n=1) with 2000 mg/day. In some patients starting with higher doses suggested that upward titration was necessary for antimanic efficacy, which is represented by table 5.10 and figure 5.9.

Table 5.10: Starting doses of SVA

Drug	Dose (mg/day)	Frequency (n)
SVA	1000	11 (36.66%)
	1500	18 (60%)
	2000	1 (3.33%)
Total		30

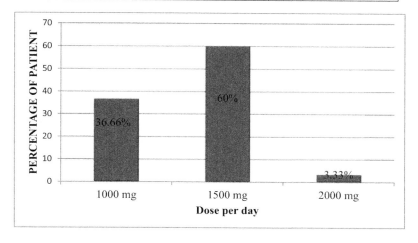

Figure 5.9: Bar diagram showing starting dose of SVA.

EFFICACY OF SVA

From 30 patients who responded, the mean baseline score for all cases treated with
SVA on day 0 using the YMRS was 38.87 ± 3.739. On day 7of the study period, the
percentage of patients who reported had YMRS scores decreased by 14.32% as in
table 5.11. Overall mean score for all cases on day 7on YMRS was 33.30 ± 2.769,
and on day 30 the score was 13.90 ± 1.954 which was significantly lower than that
compared to the baseline score on day 0 ($p= 0.00$). YMRS showed 64.24 % reduction
in mean score for all cases from day 0 to day 30 as in table 5.12.

**Table 5.11: Change in YMRS score on day 7 from baseline in patients receiving
SVA**

Day	Mean	Frequency(n)	Std. Deviation	Std. Error Mean	p- value
Day 0	38.87	30	3.739	.683	0.000*
Day 7	33.30	30	2.769	.505	

Paired-Samples t-test * Significant difference existed at $p < 0.05$.

**Table 5.12: Change in YMRS score on day 30 from baseline in patients receiving
SVA**

Day	Mean	Frequency(n)	Std. Deviation	Std. Error Mean	p- value
Day 0	38.87	30	3.739	.683	0.000*
Day 30	13.90	30	1.954	.357	

Paired-Samples t-test * Significant difference existed at $p < 0.05$.

Change in the YMRS scores of individual items with SVA:

Maximum reduction in the YMRS scale was seen with the disruptive aggressive behavior (71.08%) and minimum with insight (14.22%) over 30 days durations as depicted by table 5.13 and figure 5.10.

Table 5.13: Changes in Mean YMRS parameter scores at baseline, at day 7 and at day 30 of treatment with SVA

YMRS parameters	YMRS on day 0 (Mean ± SD)	YMRS on day 7 (Mean ± SD)	YMRS on day 30 (Mean ± SD)
Elevated mood	3.27 ± 0.521	3.13 ± 0.507	1.03 ± 0.556
Increased motor activity	2.80 ± 0.847	2.13 ± 0.629	0.43 ± 0.504
Sexual interest	2.30 ± 0.596	1.77 ± 0.430	0.13 ± 0.346
Sleep	2.87 ± 0.571	1.87 ± 0.571	0.27 ± 0.450
Irritation	4.40 ± 0.814	4.00 ± 0.743	1.60 ± 0.814
Speech	5.53 ± 1.137	4.47 ± 0.860	2.00 ± 0.000
Language thought disorder	2.53 ± 0.507	2.50 ± 0.509	1.67 ± 0.479
Content	5.40 ± 0.932	5.20 ± 0.997	2.27 ± 0.691
Disruptive aggressive behavior	4.60 ± 1.303	3.40 ± 0.932	1.33 ± 0.959
Appearance	2.70 ± 0.651	2.30 ± 0.651	1.13 ± 0.571
Insight	2.53 ± 0.507	2.53 ± 0.507	2.17 ± 0.531

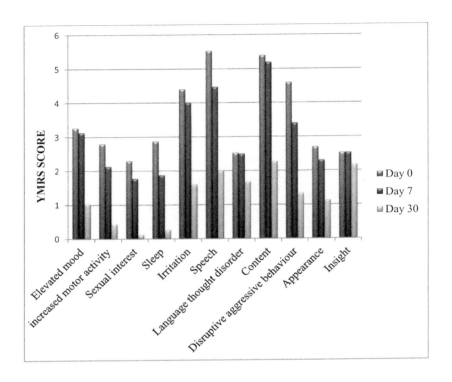

Figure 5.10: Graph showing the effects of SVA on day 0, 7 and 30.

STARTING DOSES OF OLZ

In the present study, 30 bipolar affective disorder, mania patients having different scores on the YMRS, were treated with different doses of OLZ ranging from 10 mg/day to 20 mg/day. Among them 63.33% (n=20) were started with 20 mg/day, 23.33% (n= 7) were started with 15 mg/day and 13.33% (n= 4) with 10 mg/day. In some patients starting with higher doses suggested that upward titration was necessary for antimanic efficacy, which is represented by table 5.14 and figure 5.11.

Table 5.14: Starting doses of OLZ

Drug	Dose (mg/day)	Frequency (n)
OLZ	10	4 (13.33%)
	15	7 (23.33%)
	20	19 (63.33%)
Total		30

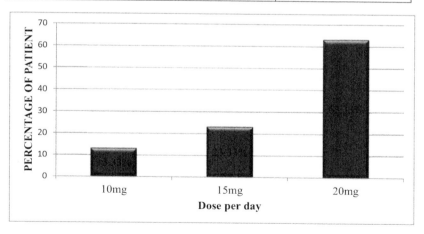

Figure 5.11: Bar diagram showing starting dose of OLZ.

49

EFFICACY OF OLZ

From 30 patients who responded, the mean baseline score for all cases treated with OLZ on day 0 using the YMRS was 40.83 ± 6.502. On day 7 of the study period, the percentage of patients who reported had YMRS scores decreased by 16.85%. Overall mean score for all cases on day 7 on YMRS was 34.03 ± 4.679 as in table 5.15 and on day 30 the score was 14.47 ± 2.837 as in table 5.16, which was significantly lower than that compared to the baseline score on day 0 (p= 0.00). YMRS showed 64.56 % reduction in mean score for all cases from day 0 to day 30.

Table 5.15: Change in YMRS score on day 7 from baseline in patients receiving OLZ

Day	Mean	Frequency(n)	Std. Deviation	Std. Error Mean	p- value
Day 0	40.83	30	6.502	1.187	0.000*
Day 7	34.03	30	4.679	.854	

Paired-Samples t-test * Significant difference existed at $p < 0.05$.

Table 5.16: Change in YMRS score on day 30 from baseline in patients receiving OLZ

Day	Mean	Frequency(n)	Std. Deviation	Std. Error Mean	p- value
Day 0	40.83	30	6.502	1.187	0.000*
Day 30	14.47	30	2.837	.518	

Paired-Samples t-test * Significant difference existed at $p < 0.05$.

Change in the YMRS scores of individual items with OLZ:

Maximum reduction in the YMRS scale was seen with the disruptive aggressive behavior (77.37%) and minimum with insight (22.29%) over 30 days durations as depicted by table 5.17 and figure 5.12.

TABLE 5.17: Changes in Mean YMRS parameter scores at baseline, at day 7 and at day 30 of treatment with OLZ

YMRS parameters	YMRS on day 0 (Mean ± SD)	YMRS on day 7 (Mean ± SD)	YMRS on day 30 (Mean ± SD)
Elevated mood	3.27 ± 0.785	3.23 ± 0.774	0.97 ± 0.556
Increased motor activity	3.07 ± 0.740	2.23 ± 0.568	0.50 ± 0.509
Sexual interest	2.27 ± 0.691	1.83 ± 0.592	0.30 ± 0.466
Sleep	3.33 ± 0.711	2.27 ± 0.691	0.37 ± 0.490
Irritation	4.60 ± 1.070	3.80 ± 1.095	1.60 ± 0.814
Speech	5.73 ± 1.143	4.67 ± 0.959	2.27 ± 0.691
Language thought disorder	2.83 ± 0.592	2.80 ± 0.610	2.03 ± 0.669
Content	5.53 ± 1.456	4.87 ± 1.252	2.20 ± 0.610
Disruptive aggressive behavior	4.73 ± 1.437	3.27 ± 0.980	1.07 ± 1.015
Appearance	2.70 ± 0.535	2.23 ± 0.568	0.97 ± 0.556
Insight	2.87 ± 0.629	2.83 ± 0.592	2.23 ± 0.504

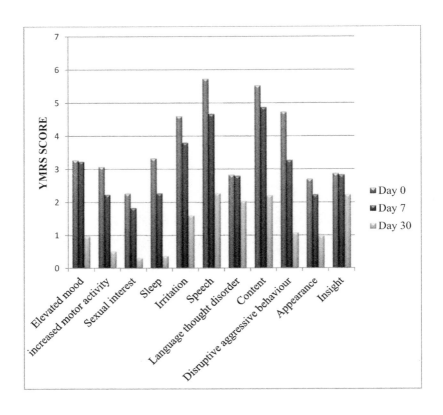

Figure 5.12: Graph showing effects of OLZ on day 0, 7 and 30.

Overall change in YMRS scores of individual items with both the drugs:

Maximum reduction in the YMRS scale was seen with the disruptive aggressive behavior (74.30%) and minimum with insight (18.51%) over 30 days durations as depicted by table 5.18 and figure 5.13.

Table 5.18: Changes in Mean YMRS parameter scores at baseline, at day 7 and at day 30 of treatment with both drug groups

YMRS parameters	YMRS on day 0 (Mean ± SD)	YMRS on day 7 (Mean ± SD)	YMRS on day 30 (Mean ± SD)
Elevated mood	3.27 ± 0.660	3.18 ± 0.651	1.00 ± 0.552
Increased motor activity	2.93 ± 0.800	2.18 ± 0.596	0.47 ± 0.503
Sexual interest	2.28 ± 0.640	1.80 ± 0.514	0.22 ± 0.415
Sleep	3.10 ± 0.681	2.07 ± 0.660	0.32 ± 0.469
Irritation	4.50 ± 0.948	3.90 ± 0.933	1.60 ± 0.807
Speech	5.63 ± 1.134	4.57 ± 0.909	2.13 ± 0.503
Language thought disorder	2.68 ± 0.567	2.65 ± 0.577	1.85 ± 0.606
Content	5.47 ± 1.214	5.03 ± 1.134	2.23 ± 0.647
Disruptive aggressive behavior	4.67 ± 1.361	3.33 ± 0.951	1.20 ± 0.988
Appearance	2.70 ± 0.591	2.27 ± 0.607	1.05 ± 0.565
Insight	2.70 ± 0.591	2.68 ± 0.567	2.20 ± 0.514

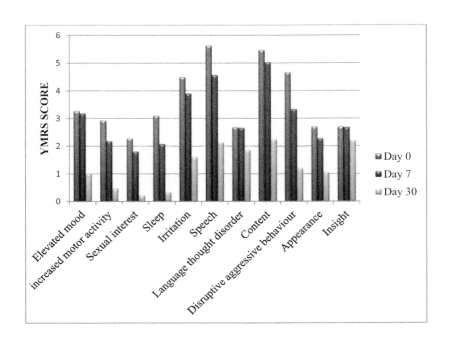

Figure 5.13: Mean scores of YMRS parameters at baseline, day 7 and at day 30 of treatment with both treatment groups.

MEAN OVERALL REDUCTION OF YMRS SCORES:

Table 5.19: Mean overall reduction in YMRS by both drugs

Drug Group	YMRS on day 0 (Mean ± SD)	YMRS on day 7 (Mean ± SD)	YMRS on day 30 (Mean ± SD)
SVA	38.87 ± 3.739	33.30 ± 2.769	13.90 ± 1.954
OLZ	40.83 ± 6.502	34.03 ± 4.679	14.47 ± 2.837

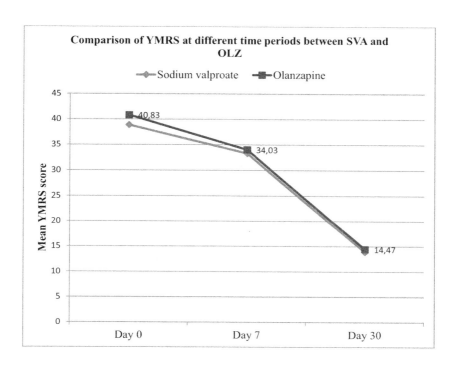

Figure 5.14: Graph showing mean YMRS score at baseline, day 7 and at day 30 of treatment with SVA and OLZ.

The mean baseline YMRS score for all cases on sodium valproate (n=30) on day 0 was 38.87 ± 3.73, 33.30 ± 2.769 on day 7 and was reduced to 13.90 ± 1.95 (p= 0.371) on day 30. Similarly, the mean baseline YMRS score for all cases on OLZ (n=30) on day 0 was 40.83 ± 6.50, 34.03 ± 4.679 on day 7 and was reduced to 14.47 ± 2.83 (p= 0.371) on day 30, as shown in table 5.19 and figure 5.14.

DISCUSSION

The present study was conducted to compare the efficacy of SVA (500-2000 mg/day) and OLZ (5-20mg/day) in the treatment of bipolar affective disorder, mania. A total of 60 patients, 18-70 years old were divided into 25 (41.7 %) and 35 (58.3 %) females. The efficacy of both the test drugs were assessed and recorded at baseline, day 7 and day 30 using Young Mania Rating Scale (YMRS).

The emphasis of the treatment of BPD, mania is on effective management of the long-term course of the illness, which can involve treatment of emergent symptoms. Treatment methods include pharmacological and psychological techniques.

The primary treatment for BPD, mania consists of medications called mood stabilizers, which are used to prevent or control episodes of mania or depression. Medications from several classes have mood stabilizing activity. Many individuals may require a combination of medication to achieve full remission of symptoms. The goal of treatment is not to cure the disorder but rather to control the symptoms and the course of the disorder.

Age: Out of the total 60 patients enrolled in the study, 30 received SVA and 30 received OLZ. The mean age of patients enrolled in the SVA group was 36.77 years while those in OLZ group was 37.40 years. The mean age of the patients in both the groups were not statistically significantly different (p= 0.312). Maximum number of patients who were treated with SVA belonged to 18-27 years (26.66%) age group and the maximum number of patients who were treated with OLZ belonged to 28 - 37 years (33.33%) age group. 21 (35%) patients were from the age group 28 - 37 years, 14 (23.33%) belonged to the age group 18 - 27 years and 38 - 47 years, 6 (10%) belonged to the age group 48-57 years, 4 (6.67%) belonged to age group 58-67 years and 1 (1.67%) belonged to 68 years and above. Age distribution was similar in both the treatment groups (p = 0.312 on Chi-square test). The mean age of patients diagnosed bipolar affective disorder, mania was 39.80 years which is similar to the mean age of studies conducted by Tohen et al.[27] and Tohen et al.[104], where 35% of the patients were in the age group of 28-37 years.

18-70 years age group distribution in this study is similar to the age group distribution of studies conducted by Tohen et al.[27], Tohen et al.[104], Tohen et al.[108], Hirschfield et al.[9], Khanna et al. , Khattri et al., where maximum patients belonged to the age group of 21-30 (25.7%) and 31-40 (24.1%) years.

Sex: Females were the predominant sex 58.3% (n=35), followed by males 41.7% (n=25) of the total study population. There was no significant difference in the sex of the patents in the two treatment groups (p= 0.793 on Chi-square test). Similar predominance of females was also seen in studies conducted by Tohen et al.[104] (female=57.4%); Tohen et al.[27] (female 57%) and Khattri et al. (females 50.4%).

Marital status: 41 (68.33%) patients were married and 19 (31.66%) patients were unmarried. On Chi-square test there was no significant statistical difference in the marital status of the patients in the both treatment groups (p= 0.781).

Religion: Out of the total patients 34 (56.66%) belonged to Hindu religion and 26 (43.33%) belonged to other religion. On Chi-square test there was no significant statistical difference in the marital status of the patients in the both treatment groups (p= 0.297).

Occupation: Out of 60 patients involved in the study 21 (35%) were housewife, 16 (26.66) were farmers, 10 (16.66%) were unemployed, 7 (11.665) were involved in business and 6 (10%) were student. There was no statistically significant difference in the occupation distribution in both the treatment groups (Chi-square test, p= 0.150).

Socioeconomic status (SES):

29 (48.33%) belonged to low SES, 22 (36.66%) belonged to middle SES and 9 (15%) belonged to the high SES group. There was no statistically significant difference in the socioeconomic status of the patients enrolled in both the treatment groups (Chi-square test, p= 0.930).

Study Design:

Tohen et al.[104] conducted a 47-week, randomized, double-blind study comparing flexibly dosed OLZ (5–20 mg/day) to DVP (500–2500 mg/day) for manic or mixed episodes of BPD. The primary efficacy instrument was the YMRS; a prioriprotocol-defined threshold scores were ≥20 for inclusion, ≤12 for remission and ≥15 for relapse. Similar drug doses and assessment scale were also used in studies conducted by Tohen et al.[27], Tohen et al.[107], Kumar et al.[15] and Niufan et al.[102]

Similarly, YMRS was also used as an assessment scale in studies conducted by Pope et al.[25], Müller-Oerlinghausen et al.[97] and Cazorla et al[101].

Other scales used for assessing mania, included Clinical Global Impression Scale for Bipolar Illness (CGI-BP), Brief Psychiatry Rating Scale (BPRS), Monthomery-Åsberg Depression Rating Scale (MADRS) by Niufan et al.[102], Mania Rating Scale (MRS) by Zajecka et al.[106], HRSG by Baker et al.[103] and HRQL by Reviki et al.[105]

In this study, the study design was similar to that conducted by Tohen et al.[104], Tohen et al.[27], Tohen et al.[107], Kumar et al.[15], Niufan et al.[102] and the assessment scale used was YMRS similar to assessment scales used by Tohen et al.[104], Tohen et al.[27], Pope et al.[25], Müller-Oerlinghausen et al.[97], Cazorla et al.[101] and Niufan et al.[102]

Doses of SVA and OLZ in this study was used similar to the doses used by the studies conducted by Tohen et al.[104], Tohen et al.[107], Kumar et al.[15] and Niufan et al.[102]

DURATION OF ASSESSMENT:

The duration of assessment of this study was similar to the study duration of studies conducted by Niufan et al.[102] (4 weeks), Cazorla et al.[101] (3 week), Kumar et al.[15] (3 week), Ozcan et al.[96] (3 week), Tohen et al.[27] (3 week). However the study assessment duration was longer for studies conducted by Tohen et al.[104] (47 week), Zajecka et al.[106] (12 week), Baker et al.[103] (6 week), Tariot et al.[95] (6 week), Tohen et al.[107] (18 months), Tohen et al.[108] (6 week) and Reviki et al.[105] (12 weeks).

Sample size:

The sample size in this study was 60 which was more than that of Pope et al.[25] (n=36), Kumar et al.[15] (n=30), but less than that of Baker et al.[103] (n=85), Niufan et al.[102] (n=140), Kim et al.[112] (n=179), Osso et al.[111] (n=108), Tohen et al.[104] (n=251), Tohen et al.[27] (n =248) and Cazorla et al.[101] (n=977).

SVA as an Antimanic agent: Studies

In an open label clinical comparative study by Ozcan et al.[96] VLP reduced assessment scale scores significantly at the end of third week, showing VLP as an efficacious antimanic agent with no superiority in treatment of mania to Li and CBZ.

Similarly, a placebo-controlled, double-blind study by Pope et al.[25] on VLP in the treatment of acute mania, reported that VLP proved to be superior to placebo in alleviating manic symptoms and concluded that VLP represents a useful new drug for the treatment of manic patients.

Also in a pooled analysis, from 3 randomized, double-blind, parallel-group, active- or placebo-controlled studies, it was found that the oral loading of DVP leads to a more rapid antimanic effect and that DVP is better tolerated than OLZ.[9]

Similarly in a study on treatment of mania, mixed state and rapid cycling to summarize the quality of evidence for the efficacy of different biological treatments in mania, DVP sodium was effective in classical pure mania, whereas DVP sodium and CBZ were likely more effective in mixed states.[98]

Another 6-week, multicenter, randomized, double-blind, placebo-controlled, parallel-group study by Tariot et al.[95] showed that VLP improved symptoms of agitation.

OLZ as an Antimanic agent: Studies

Poo et al.[100] study to review the efficacy and tolerability profiles of atypical antipsychotics used to treat adult BPD in clinical practice, concluded that OLZ monotherapy was useful in the management of adult BPD in the subsets of mania, depression or mixed episodes. OLZ had anti-manic effects and it also demonstrated anti-depressant features.

Similarly, a multicenter, double-blind, randomized, controlled trial by Niufan et al.[102] on OLZ versus Li in the acute treatment of bipolar mania, the rate of response was significantly greater in the OLZ treatment group compared to the Li group.

An exploratory post hoc, pooled analysis by Cazorla et al.[101], showed that each of the eleven individual YMRS item scores was significantly reduced by asenapine and OLZ compared with placebo at day 21. After 2 days of treatment, asenapine and OLZ were superior to placebo for six of the YMRS items: disruptive/aggressive behavior, content, irritability, elevated mood, sleep and speech.

Similarly, a systematic literature review on OLZ in Chinese patients with schizophrenia or BPD, showed statistically significant reductions in symptom measures in studies conducted for $\geq$ 6 weeks (schizophrenia) or $\geq$ 3 weeks (BPD) in Chinese population.[99]

Efficacy of SVA versus OLZ:

Change in total YMRS scores from baseline (day 0) to day 7 and day 30 after intervention with SVA and OLZ was significantly changed showing that both the drugs are effective in reducing the psychopathology.

Both SVA and OLZ were as effective as each other in the 12 week multicenter study conducted by Zajecka eta al.[106] Also in the review of OLZ in management of acute mania done by Narsimhan et al.[12] showed equal efficacy of both the drugs.

Similarly, a 12-week, double-blind, double-dummy, randomized clinical trial by Reviki et al.[105] showed that DVP and OLZ have similar short-term effects on clinical or HRQL outcomes in BPD subjects.

Also, a multiple-treatments meta-analysis by Cipriani et al.[109] on comparative efficacy and acceptability of antimanic drugs in acute mania showed that OLZ was more effective than VLP. However, OLZ (standardised mean difference [SMD] -0·43 [95% CI -0·54 to -0·32]) and VLP (-0·20 [-0·37 to -0·04]) were significantly more effective than placebo.

However, the findings in this study are in contradiction to the studies conducted by Tohen et al.[104] and Tohen et al.[27], which suggest that OLZ had a greater efficacy than SVA in treatment of BPD, mania.

Similarly there are also studies which support the use of combination therapy of SVA and OLZ in the treatment of BPD, mania. Studies conducted by Baker et al.[103], Tohen et al.[108], Bai et al.[110], Kumar et al.[15] and Tohen et al.[107] suggested that the use of combination therapy had a greater efficacy in reduction of rating scores of mania.

Individual items in YMRS:

In this study, out of the 11 items of YMRS, maximum reduction was seen in the item disruptive aggressive behavior (71.08%) and minimum reduction was seen in insight (14.22%) from baseline to day 30 with SVA (TG1). Similarly for OLZ group (TG2) maximum reduction was seen in disruptive aggressive behavior (26.08%) with no reduction in insight.

Overall, the highest reduction was seen in disruptive aggressive behavior (74.30%) and minimum reduction was seen in insight (18.51%) from baseline to day 30 in both the treatment groups, which is consistent with the findings of studies conducted by Cazorla et al.[101], Tohen et al.[104] and Pope et al.[25]

LIMITATIONS AND FUTURE DIRECTIONS

The limitations of the present study should also be considered along with analyzing the result.

- Relatively low number of cases (n=60), short duration of assessment and a single site of study made it difficult to generalize the results to other medical centers and the entire Nepalese population.
- All patients with BPD, mania were not enrolled. Enrollment was based on willingness of patient relatives, patient themselves and co-operation of on duty Psychiatrist.
- A single scale for assessment was used.
- Adverse effects, cost of drug was not taken into consideration.

An area of potential further studies would be to use larger sample size, longer duration of assessment in hospitals of different levels including community health centers along with the use of a placebo arm in this study.

Further research would benefit from more prospective randomized controlled trials evaluating the efficacy of existing and newer atypical antipsychotics and different combinations of drug regimens in order to maximize clinical benefit and minimizing adverse events. The assessment of established atypical antipsychotics could also be trialed on different subgroups of patients.

Despite its limitations, present study is a longitudinal study which is better than cross sectional study. In the present study, the antimanic efficacy is compared in three visits, allowing close monitoring of the effects of both the drugs in patients.

SUMMARY AND CONCLUSION

This study entitled "A comparative study on efficacy of sodium valproate and olanzapine in the patients of Bipolar affective disorder, mania in CMS-TH, Bharatpur." is a longitudinal (prospective) study. The present study was conducted at Department of Psychiatry of College of Medical Sciences Teaching Hospital. In the present study, as assessed by YMRS score, both sodium valproate and olanzapine were effective antimanic drugs (i.e., significantly lower mean YMRS score; $p < 0.05$) at day 0, 7 and 30. Overall, the mean decrease in YMRS score was 64.41%, (decrease in YMRS score by sodium valproate was 64.24% and with olanzapine was 64.56%).

CONCLUSION

As evident from the present study, both the drugs show significant mean improvement of mania ratings in both the treatment groups. Likewise, the findings of the present study are comparable with other studies and can be used as supportive evidence for further studies. Thus, this study shows that sodium valproate and olanzapine has no statistically significant difference in efficacy in treatment of bipolar affective disorder, mania.

REFERENCES:

1.   American Psychiatric Association. Diagnostic and statistical manual of mental disorders. 4th ed. Washington DC: American Psychiatric Association; 2000.

2.   World Health Organization. The ICD-10 Classification of mental and behavioural disorders. Geneva: World Health Organisation; 1992.

3.   Schaffer A, Cairney J, Cheung A, Veldhuizen S, Levitt A. Community survey of bipolar disorder in Canada: lifetime prevalence and illness characteristics. Can J Psychiatry 2006;51:9-16.

4.   Goodwin FK, Jamison KR, editors. Manic-depressive illness: bipolar and recurrent depression. 2nd ed. New York: Oxford University Press; 2007.

5.   World Health Organization. The International statistical classification of diseases and related health problems. Geneva: WHO Press; 2004.

6.   Blader JC, KafantarisV. Pharmacological treatment of bipolar disorder among children and adolescents. Expert Rev Neurother 2007;7(3):259–70.

7.   Spearing M. Bipolar Disorder. 2nd ed. Bethesda (MA): National institute of mental health; 2001.21(4).360-68.

8.   McDonald WM, Wermager J. Pharmacologic treatment of geriatric mania. Current Psychiatry Reports 2002; 4(1):43-50.

9.   Hirschfeld RM, Baker JD, Wozniak P, Tracy K, Sommerville KW. The safety and early efficacy of oral-loaded divalproex versus standard-titration divalproex, lithium, olanzapine, and placebo in the treatment of acute mania associated with bipolar disorder. J Clin Psychiatry 2003;64(7):841-6.

10.   Angst J. The emerging epidemiology of hypomania and bipolar II disorder. Journal of Affective Disorders 1998;50:143-51.

11. Derry S, Moore RA. Atypical antipsychotics in bipolar disorder: systematic review of randomised trials. BMC Psychiatry 2007;7:40.

12. Narasimhan M, Bruce TO, Masand P. Review of olanzapine in the management of bipolar disorders. Neuropsychiatric Disease and Treatment 2007;3(5):579–87.

13. Bridle C, Palme S, Bagnall A-M, Darba J, Duffy S, Sculpher M, Riemsma R. A rapid and systematic review and economic evaluation of the clinical and cost-effectiveness of newer drugs for treatment of mania associated with bipolar affective disorder. Health Technology Assessment 2004;8(19):1-97.

14. Silpakit C, Silpakit O. A review of carbamazepine and valproate use in a psychiatric hospital in Thailand. ASEAN Journal of Psychiatry 2007;8(1):9-14.

15. Kumar A, Gupta M, Jiloha RC, Tekur U. Efficacy of olanzapine and sodium valproate given alone or as add-on therapy in acute mania. A comparative study. Methods Find Exp Clin Pharmacol 2010;32(5):319-24.

16. Yatham LN, Grossman F, Augustyns I, Vieta E, Ravindran A. Mood stabilisers plus risperidone or placebo in the treatment of acute mania. International, double-blind, randomised controlled trial. Br J Psychiatry 2003;182:141-7.

17. Bowden CL. Treatment options in bipolar disorder: mood stabilizers. Medscape Psychiatry and Mental Health Journal 1997;2(4):1-6.

18. Ketter TA, Wang PW, Becker OV, Nowakowska C, Yang YS. The diverse roles of anticonvulsants in bipolar disorders. Annals of Clinical Psychiatry 2003;15(2):95-6.

19. Citrome L, Casey DE, Daniel DG, Wozniak P, Kochan LD, Tracy KA. Adjunctive divalproex and hostility among patients with schizophrenia receiving olanzapine or risperidone. Psychiatr Serv 2004;55(3):290-4.

20. Donovan SJ, Stewart JW, Nunes EV, Quitkin FM, Parides M, Daniel W, et al. Divalproex treatment for youth with explosive temper and mood lability: a double-blind, placebo-controlled crossover design. Am J Psychiatry 2000;157(5):818-20.

21. Bowden CL, Brugger AM, Swann AC, Calabrese JR, Janicak PG, Petty F, et al. Efficacy of divalproex vs lithium and placebo in the treatment of mania. The Depakote Mania Study Group. JAMA 1994;271(12):918-24.

22. Bowden CL, Calabrese JR, McElroy SL, Gyulai L, Wassef A, Petty F, et al. A randomized, placebo-controlled 12-month trial of divalproex and lithium in treatment of outpatients with bipolar I disorder. Divalproex maintenance study Group. Arch Gen Psychiatry 2000;57(5):481-9.

23. Calabrese JR, Shelton MD, Rapport DJ, Youngstrom EA, Jackson K, Bilali S, et al. A 20-month, double-blind, maintenance trial of lithium versus divalproex in rapid-cycling bipolar disorder. Am J Psychiatry 2005;162(11):2152-61.

24. Davis LL, Bartolucci A, Petty F. Divalproex in the treatment of bipolar depression: a placebo-controlled study. J Affect Disord 2005;85(3):259-66.

25. Pope HG, McElroy SL, Keck PE, Hudson JI. Valproate in the treatment of acute mania. A placebo-controlled study. Arch Gen Psychiatry 1991;48(1):62-8.

26. Sachs G, Chengappa KN, Suppes T, Mullen JA, Brecher M, Devine NA, Sweitzer DE. Quetiapine with lithium or divalproex for the treatment of bipolar mania: a randomized, double-blind, placebo-controlled study. Bipolar Disord 2004;6(3):213-23.

27. Tohen M, Baker RW, Altshuler LL, Zarate CA, Suppes T, Ketter TA, et al. Olanzapine versus divalproex in the treatment of acute mania. Am J Psychiatry 2002;159(6):1011-7.

28. Welge JA, Keck PE, Meinhold JM. Predictors of response to treatment of acute bipolar manic episodes with divalproex sodium or placebo in 2 randomized, controlled, parallel group trials. J Clin Psychopharmacol 2004;24(6):607-12.

29. Bowden CL, Swann AC, Calabrese JR, Rubenfaer LM, Wozniak PJ, Collins MA, et al. A randomized, placebo controlled, multicenter study of divalproex sodium extended release in the treatment of acute mania. J Clin Psychiatry 2006;67(10):1501-10.

30. Freeman TW, Clothier JL, Pazzaglia P, Lesem MD, Swann AC. A double-blind comparison of valproate and lithium in the treatment of acute mania. Am J Psychiatry 1992;149(1):108-11.

31. Calabrese JR, Woyshville MJ, Kimmel SE, Rapport DJ. Predictors of valproate response in bipolar rapid cycling. J Clin Psychopharmacol 1993;13(4):280-3.

32. McDonald WM, Nemeroff CB. The diagnosis and treatment of mania in the elderly. Bull Menninger Clin 1996;60:174-96.

33. Worrel JA, Marken PA, Beckman SE, Ruehter VL. Atypical antipsychotic agents: a critical review. Am J Health-Syst Pharm 2000;57:238-58.

34. Bymaster FP, Calligaro DO, Falcone JF, Marsh RD, Moore NA, Tye NC, et al. Radioreceptor binding profile of the atypical antipsychotic olanzapine. Neuropsychopharmacology 1996;14:87–96.

35. Rendell JM, Gijsman HJ, Keck P, Goodwin GM, Geddes JR. Olanzapine alone or in combination for acute mania. Cochrane Database Syst Rev. 2003;3:46-87.

36. Allison DB, Mentore JL, Heo M, Chandler LP, Cappelleri JC, Infante MC, Weiden PJ. Antipsychotic-induced weight gain: a comprehensive research synthesis. Am J Psychiatry 1999;156:1686–96.

37. Swann AC. What is bipolar disorder? Am J Psychiatry 2006;163:177-9.

38. Perlis RH, Ostacher MJ, Patel JK, Marangell LB, Zhang H, Wisniewski SR, et al. Predictors of recurrence in bipolar disorder: primary outcomes from the systematic treatment enhancement program for bipolar disorder (STEP-BD). Am J Psychiatry 2006;163:217-24.

39. Johnson SL. Defining bipolar disorder. In S. L. Johnson's (Ed.) Psychological treatments of bipolar disorder. New York: The Guilford Press. 2004;p. 3-16.

40. Pichot P. The birth of bipolar disorder. European Psychiatry 1995;10(1):1-10.

41. Angst J and Marneros A. Bipolarity from ancient to modern times: conception, birth and rebirth. Journal of Affective Disorders 2001;67:3-19.

42. Healy D. Mania: A short history of bipolar disorder. Baltimore: The John Hopkins University Press. 2008;3-4.

43. Ackerknecht EH. A short history of psychiatry. Second edition. Translated by Wolff S. New York: Hafner Publishing Company.1968;p.15.

44. American Psychiatric Association. Diagnostic and statistical manual of mental disorders. Third edition (DSM-III). Washington, DC: American Psychiatric Association.1980.

45. World Health Organization. Manual of international statistical classification of diseases, injuries and causes of death, Ninth Revision. Vol.1. Geneva: World Health Organization. 1977.

46. American Psychiatric Association. Diagnostic and statistical manual of mental disorders. Third edition –Revised (DSM-III-R). Washington DC: American Psychiatric Association. 1987.

47. American Psychiatric Association. Diagnostic and statistical manual of mental disorders. Fourth edition. International version (DSM-IV). Washington DC: American Psychiatric Association. 1995.

48. American Psychiatric Association. Diagnostic and statistical manual of mental disorders. Fifth edition (DSM-5). Washington DC: American Psychiatric Association. 2013.

49. Liddell HG, Scott R. A Greek-English Lexicon, on Perseus Digital Library.

50. Berrios GE. "Of mania". History of psychiatry. 2004;15(57 Pt 1):105–124.

51. Semple, David. "Oxford hand book of psychiatry" Oxford press, 2005.p.238.

52. Johnson SL. & Meyer B. Psychosocial predictors of symptoms. In S. L. Johnson's (Ed.) Psychological Treatments of bipolar disorder. New York: The Guilford Press. 2004;17-34.

53. Akiskal HS, Bourgeois ML, Angst J, Post R, Moller HJ, Hirschfeld RMA. Re-evaluating the prevalence of and diagnostic composition within the broad clinical spectrum of bipolar disorders. Journal of Affective Disorders 2000; 59(1),5-30.

54. Judd LL, Akiskal HS. The prevalence and disability of bipolar spectrum disorders in the U.S. population: re-analysis of the ECA database taking into account sub threshold cases. Journal of Affective Disorder 2003;73:123-131.

55. NAMI. "The many faces and facets of BP". Psychopharmacology Bulletin 2007; 32(1):55-61.Retrieved 2008-10-02.

56. Giannini AJ. Biological foundations of clinical psychiatry, NY Medical Examination Publishing Company.1986.

57. Ytham LN, Kusumakar V, Kutchar SP. (2002). Bipolar disorder: A clinician's guide to biological treatments. 2002;p.3.

58. Fletcher K, Parker G, Paterson A, Synnott H. "High-risk behaviour in hypomanic states". J Affect Disord 2013;150(1):50–6.

59. Baldessarini RJ, Tarazi FI. Pharmacotherapy of psychosis and mania.In Goodman, Brunton L, Chabner B, Knollman B, editor. Goodman Gilman's pharmacological basis of therapeutics. 12th ed. New York: McGraw-Hill Professional. 2011.p.301-20.

60. Li X, Liu M, Cai Z, Wang G, Li X. "Regulation of glycogen synthase kinase-3 during bipolar mania treatment". Bipolar Disord 2010;2(7):741–52.

61. Yildiz A, Guleryuz S, Ankerst DP, Ongür D, Renshaw PF. "Protein kinase C inhibition in the treatment of mania: a double-blind, placebo-controlled trial of tamoxifen". Arch. Gen. Psychiatry 2008;65(3):255–63.

62. Brietzke E, Stertz L, Fernandes BS, Kauer-Sant'anna M, Mascarenhas M, Escosteguy VA, Chies JA, Kapczinski F. "Comparison of cytokine levels in depressed, manic and euthymic patients with bipolar disorder". J Affect Disord 2009;116(3):214–7.

63. Altshuler L, Bookheimer S, Proenza MA, Townsend J, Sabb F, Firestine A, Bartzokis G, Mintz J, Mazziotta J, Cohen MS. "Increased amygdala activation during mania: a functional magnetic resonance imaging study". Am J Psychiatry 2005;162(6):1211–13.

64. Gelder M, Mayou R, Geddes J. Psychiatry. 3rd edition. Oxford: Oxford University Press. 2006.p.105.

65. Loscher W. Basic pharmacology of valproate: a review after 35 years of clinical use for the treatment of epilepsy. CNS Drugs. 2002;16:669–94.

66. Casey DE, Daniel DG, Wassef AA, Tracy KA, Wozniak P, Sommerville KW. Effect of divalproex combined with olanzapine or risperidone in patients with an acute exacerbation of schizophrenia. Neuropsychopharmacol 2003;28:182–92.

71

67. Post RM. Mood disorders: Treatment of Bipolar disorder. In: Sadock BJ, Sadock VA, editor. Kaplan and Sadock's comprehensive textbook of psychiatry. 7th ed. New York: Lippincott Williams and Wilkins Publishers; 2000.p.2779-870.

68. Toth M. The epsilon theory: a novel synthesis of the underlying molecular and electrophysiological mechanisms of primary generalized epilepsy and the possible mechanism of action of valproate. Medical Hypotheses. 2005;64:267–72.

69. Owens MJ, Nemeroff CB. Pharmacology of valproate. Psychopharmacology Bulletin. 2003;37(Suppl 2):S17–24.

70. Harwood AJ, Agam G. Search for a common mechanism of mood stabilizers. Biochemical Pharmacology. 2003;66:179–89.

71. Shaltiel G, Shamir G, Shapiro J. Valproate decreases inositol biosynthesis. Biological Psychiatry. 2004;56:868–74.

72. Olanzapine Prescribing Information" (PDF). Eli Lilly and Company. 2009:1-34.

73. "Bipolar disorder: the assessment and management of bipolar disorder in adults, children and young people in primary and secondary care. NICE guidelines (CG185), 2014. Available from http://www.nice.org.uk/guidance/cg185/chapter/1recommendations.html

74. Yatham LN, Kennedy SH, O'Donovan C, Parikh SV, MacQueen G, McIntyre RS, Sharma V, Beaulieu S; Guidelines Group, CANMAT. "Canadian network for mood and anxiety treatments (CANMAT) guidelines for the management of patients with bipolar disorder: update 2007". Bipolar Disord 2006;8(6):721–39.

75. Osser DN, Roudsari MJ, Manschreck T . "The psychopharmacology algorithm project at the Harvard South Shore Program: an update on schizophrenia". Harv Rev Psychiatry 2013;21(1):18–40.

76. Review of olanzapine in the management of bipolar disorders. Neuropsychiatr Dis Treat. 2007;3(5):579–587.

77. Bakshi VP, Geyer MA. Antagonism of phencyclidine-induced deficits in prepulse inhibition by the putative atypical antipsychotic olanzapine. Psychopharmacol (Berl) 1995;122(2):198-201.

78. Coyle JT. The glutamatergic dysfunction hypothesis for schizophrenia. Harv. Rev. Psychiatry 1996;3(5):241-53.

79. Fuller RW and Snoddy HD. Neuroendocrine evidence for antagonism of serotonin and dopamine receptors by olanzapine (LY170053), an antipsychotic drug candidate. Res. Commun. Chem. Pathol. Pharmacol.1992;77(1):87-93.

80. Saller CF and Salama AI. Seroquel: biochemical profile of a potential atypical antipsychotic. Psychopharmacol(Berl) 1993;112(2-3):285-92.

81. White FJ, Wang RY. Differential effects of classical and atypical antipsychotic drugs on A9 and A10 dopamine neurons. Science. 1983;221(4615):1054-57.

82. Fumagalli F, Frasca A, Sparta M, Drago F, Racagni G, Riva MA. Longterm exposure to the atypical antipsychotic olanzapine differently upregulates extracellular signal-regulated kinases 1 and 2 phosphorylation in subcellular compartments of rat prefrontal cortex. Mol Pharmacol. 2006;69(4):1366–72.

83. Kassahun K, Mattiuz E, Nyhart E Jr, Obermeyer B, Gillespie T, Murphy A, Goodwin RM, Tupper D, Callaghan JT, Lemberger L. Disposition and biotransformation of the antipsychotic agent olanzapine in humans. Drug Metab Dispos 1997;25(1):81–93.

84. Kando JC, Shepski JC, Satterlee W, Patel JK, Reams SG, Green AI. Olanzapine: a new antipsychotic agent with efficacy in the management of schizophrenia. Ann Pharmacother 1997;31(11):1325–34.

85. Aichhorn W, Weiss U, Marksteiner J, Kemmler G, Walch T, Zernig G, Stelzig-Schoeler R, Stuppaeck C, Geretsegger C. Age and gender effects on olanzapine and risperidone plasma concentrations in children and adolescents. J Child Adolesc Psychopharmacol 2007;17(5):665–74.

86. Templeman LA, Reynolds GP, Arranz B, San L. Polymorphisms of the 5-HT2C receptor and leptin genes are associated with antipsychotic drug-induced weight gain in Caucasian subjects with a first-episode psychosis. Pharmacogenet Genomics. 2005;15(4):195–200.

87. Gunes A, Melkersson KI, Scordo MG, Dahl ML. Association between HTR2C and HTR2A polymorphisms and metabolic abnormalities in patients treated with olanzapine or clozapine. J Clin Psychopharmacol 2009;29(1):65–68.

88. Wirshing DA, Wirshing WC, Kysar L, Berisford MA, Goldstein D, Pashdag J, Mintz J, Marder SR. Novel antipsychotics: comparison of weight gain liabilities. J Clin Psychiatry 1999;60(6):358–63.

89. Lexi-Comp Inc. Lexi-Comp drug information handbook 19th North American Ed. Hudson, OH: Lexi-Comp Inc. 2010.

90. WebMD [Internet]. Symbyax (Olanzapine and fluoxetine) drug overdose and contraindication information. RxList: The internet drug index. 2007;175(3):389-90.

91. Lucas RA, Gilfillan DJ, Bergstrom RF. A pharmacokinetic interaction between carbamazepine and olanzapine: observations on possible mechanism. Eur J Clin Pharmacol 1998;54(8):639–643.

92. Callaghan JT, Bergstrom RF, Ptak LR, Beasley CM. Olanzapine. Pharmacokinetic and pharmacodynamic profile. Clin Pharmacokinet. 1999;37(3):177–193.

93. Spina E, de Leon J. Metabolic drug interactions with newer antipsychotics: a comparative review. Basic Clin Pharmacol Toxicol 2007;100(1):4–22.

94. Montgomery S, van Zwieten-Boot B, Angst J, Bowden CL, Calabrese JR, Chengappa R, et al. ECNP Consensus meeting march 2000 Nice: guidelines for investigating efficacy in bipolar disorder. Eur Neuropsychopharmacol 2001;11:79–88.

95. Tariot PN, Schneider LS, Mintzer JE, Cutler AJ, Cunningham MR, Thomas JW, Sommerville KW. Safety and tolerability of divalproex sodium in the treatment of signs and symptoms of mania in elderly patients with dementia: results of a double-blind, placebo-controlled trial. 2001;62(1):51-67.

96. Ozcan M, Boztepe AV. Lithium, carbamazepine and valproate in acute mania. Bull Clin Psychopharmacol 2001;11:90-95.

97. Müller-Oerlinghausen B, Retzow A, Henn FA, Giedke H, Walden J. Valproate as an adjunct to neuroleptic medication for the treatment of acute episodes of mania: a prospective, randomized, double-blind, placebo-controlled, multicenter study. European Valproate Mania Study Group. J Clin Psychopharmacol 2000;20(2):195-203.

98. Kusumakar V, Yatham L N, Haslam D R S, Parikh S V, Matte R, Silverstone P H, Sharma V. Treatment of mania, mixed state and rapid cycling. Can J Psychiatry 1997;42(2):79S–86S.

99. Xue HBH, Liu L, Zhang H, Montgomery W, Treuer T. Olanzapine in Chinese patients with schizophrenia or bipolar disorder: a systematic literature review. Neuropsychiatric Disease and Treatment 2014;10:841–64.

100. Poo SXW, Agius M atypical anti-psychotics in adult bipolar disorder: current evidence and updates in the nice guidelines. Psychiatria Danubina 2014;26(1):322–29.

101. Cazorla P, Zhao J, Mackle M, Szegedi A. Asenapine effects on individual Young mania rating scale items in bipolar disorder patients with acute manic or mixed episodes: a pooled analysis. Neuropsychiatric Disease and Treatment 2013;9:409-13.

102. Niufan G, Tohen M, Qiuqing A, Fude Y, Pope E, McElroy H, Ming L, Gaohua W, Xinbao Z, Huichun L, Liang S. Olanzapine versus lithium in the acute treatment of bipolar mania: a double-blind, randomized, controlled trial. Journal of Affective Disorders 2008;105:101–8.

103. Baker RW, Brown E, Akiskal HS, Calabrese JR, Ketter TA, Schuh LM, et al. Efficacy of olanzapine combined with valproate or lithium in the treatment of dysphoric mania. British Journal of Psychiatry 2004;185:472–78.

104. Tohen M, Ketter TA, Zarate CA, Suppes T, Frye M, Altshuler L, et al. Olanzapine versus divalproex sodium for the treatment of acute mania and maintenance of remission: a 47-week study. Am J Psychiatry 2003;160(7):1263-71.

105. Revicki DA, Paramore LC, Sommerville KW, Swann AC, Zajecka JM. Depakote Comparator Study Group. Divalproex sodium versus olanzapine in the treatment of acute mania in bipolar disorder: health-related quality of life and medical cost outcomes. J Clin Psychiatry 2003;64(3):288-94.

106. Zajecka JM, Weisler R, Sachs G, Swann AC, Wozniak P, Sommerville KW. A comparison of the efficacy, safety, and tolerability of divalproex sodium and

olanzapine in the treatment of bipolar disorder. J Clin Psychiatry 2002;63:1148-55.

107. Tohen M, Chengappa KN, Suppes T, Baker RW, Zarate CA, Bowden CL, et al. Relapse prevention in bipolar I disorder: 18-month comparison of olanzapine plus mood stabilizer vs. mood stabiliser alone. British Journal of Psychiatry 2004;184:337–45.

108. Tohen M, Chengappa KN, Suppes T, Zarate CA, Bowden CL, Sachs GS, et al. Efficacy of olanzapine in combination with valproate or lithium in the treatment of mania in patients partially nonresponsive to valproate or lithium monotherapy. Arch Gen Psychiatry 2002;59:62–9.

109. Cipriani, A., Barbui, C., Salanti, G., Rendell, J., Brown, R., Stockton, S., Purgato, M., Spineli, L.M., Goodwin, G.M., Geddes, J.R., 2011. Comparative efficacy and acceptability of antimanic drugs in acute mania: a multiple treatments meta-analysis. Lancet. 2011;378 (9799),1306–15.

110. Bai YM, Chang CJ, Tsai SY, Cheng YC, Hsiao MC, Li CT, Tu P, Chang SW, Shen WW, Su TP. Taiwan consensus of pharmacological treatment for bipolar disorder. Journal of the Chinese Medical Association 2013;76(10):547-56.

111. Dell'Osso B, Buoli M, Riccardo Riundi, D'Urso N, Pozzoli S, Bassetti R, Mundo E, Altamura AC. Clinical characteristics and long-term response to mood stabilizers in patients with bipolar disorder and different age at onset. Neuropsychiatric Disease and Treatment. 2009;5:399–404.

112. Kim B, Kim S-J, Son J-I, Joo YH. Weight change in the acute treatment of bipolar I disorder: a naturalistic observational study of psychiatric inpatients. Journal of Affective Disorders 2008;105:45–52.

113. Luca M, Prossimo G, Messina V, Luca A, Romeo S, Calandra C. Epidemiology and treatment of mood disorders in a day hospital setting from 1996 to 2007: an Italian study . Neuropsychiatric Disease and Treatment. 2013;9:169–76.

114. Young RC, Biggs JT, Ziegler VE, Meyer DA. A rating scale for mania: reliability, validity and sensitivity. British Journal of Psychiatry 1978;133:429-35.

115. Beigel A, Murphy DL & Bunney WE. The manic-state rating scale. Archives of General Psychiatry. 1971;25:256-61

116. Altman E. Differential diagnosis and assessment of adult bipolar disorder. In S. L. Johnson's (Ed.) psychological treatment of bipolar disorder. New York: The Guildford Press. 2004;p.35-57.

sn]h ckm d]l8sn ;fO{G;];\ -lzÔ0f c:ktfn_

e/tk'/, lrtjg, g]kfn

ldlt M

d~h'/Lgfdf

==================c~rn==================

======lhNnf==================uf=lj=;=÷g=kf=j8

fg+========a:g]

==============================sf] gflt ÷

gfltgL==============================sf] ÷sf] ;f]

5f]/f÷f÷5f]/L/L÷kTgL L==============================

=======aif{========nfO{==============================

=======/f]unfu]sf] lrlsT;x?af6 yfxf x'g cfPsf]n] / ;f] /f]usf]

pkrfry{ cfjZos hf+r ljlw=========================u/fpg d

sn]h ckm d]l8sn ;fO{G;];\ e/tk'/ lrtjgdf u/fpg d~h'/L 5'.

pQm hf+rsf] af/]df lrlsT;;n] dnfO{ k'0f{{ hfgsf/L lbO{ ;]sf] / hf+r ljlwnfO{ cg]';Gwfg ug{sf] nflu k|of]u u/]dnfO{ s'g} cfklt gePsf] x'gfn] d d~h'/Lgfdf ub{5'.

la/fdLsf] gft]bf/sf] ;lx ÷5fk   x:tflf/÷cf}7f 5fk

gfd M

7]ufgf M

gftf M

d 8f= nf]s]Zj/ rf}/l;of dfly pNn]lvt hfgsf/L uf]Ko /fVg] 5' /
o;nfO{ k"0f{tof cWoogsfo{sf nfludfq k|of]u ug]{5'.

==============================

8f= nf]s]Zj/ rf}/l;of

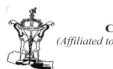

International Society for Medical Education Pvt. Ltd.
COLLEGE OF MEDICAL SCIENCES -NEPAL
(Affiliated to the Kathmandu University and Recognized by Nepal Medical Council)
P.O. Box No: 23, Bharatpur, Chitwan (Dist.), Nepal

Date:......................

INFORMED CONSENT

........................…..........Zone........................…........District..................….............

V.D.C./Municipality   Ward   No.......... Resident............. of   grandson/ granddaughter...........................of   son/daughter/wife......................of age...... have been well informed about the illnesses and diseases about the patient by the doctors. Hence, the undersigned is agreed to continue ....for necessary treatment of the patient in the College of Medical Sciences Teaching Hospital, Bharatpur, Chitwan (Dist.), Nepal.

The doctors have given me all informations regarding the treatment and investigations of the patient. Therefore, the undersigned has given the written consent that there is no objection regarding necessary treatment and investigations of the patient.

Signature/Thumb Impression of relative   Signature/Thumb Impression of patient

Name:

Address:

Relation:

I Dr. Lokeshwar Chaurasia will keep the above mentioned information confidential and sole use for research purpose.

....

Dr. Lokeshwar Chaurasia

CASE PROFORMA

Date:

Name: IP number:

Age: Sex:

Address:

Occupation: Ethnic group:

Date of examination:

Chief Complaints:

History of Presenting Illness:

Past Drug History:

Past Psychiatric History:

Medical History:

Personal History:

Family History:

History of Allergy:

Premorbid personality:

General Examination:

    Blood Pressure:

    Temperature:

    Pulse:

    Respiratory Rate:

General physical examination:

    Jaundice: Anaemia:

    Lymphadenopathy: Cyanosis :

    Clubbing: Odema:

    Dehydration:

Systemic Examination:

    Chest: CVS:

    PA: CNS:

Mental state examination:

1. General appearance, behaviour, eye contact and rapport

2. Speech

3. Mood

4. Thought form

5. Thought content

6. Perception

7. Attention and concentration

8. Memory

9. Orientation

10. General knowledge

11. Intelligence

12. Judgement

13. Insight

A. YMRS score for patients on Tab. SVA :

Baseline (day 0)	Day 7	Day 30

B. YMRS score for patients on Tab. OLZ :

Baseline (day 0)	Day 7	Day 30

Young Mania Rating Scale (YMRS)

Enter the appropriate score which best characterizes the subject for each item.

ITEM	EXPLANATION
1. Elevated mood	0 absent 1 mildly or possibly increased on questioning 2 definite subjective elevation: optimistic, self-confident; cheerful;appropriate to content 3 elevated, inappropriate to content; humorous 4 euphoric, inappropriate laughter singing
2. Increased motor activity-energy	0 absent 1 subjectively increased 2 animated; gestures increased 3 excessive energy; hyperactive at times; restless (can be calmed) 4 motor excitement; continues hyperactivity (cannot be calmed)
3. Sexual interest	0 normal; not increased 1 mildly or possibly increased 2 definite subjective increase on questioning 3 spontaneous sexual content; elaborates on sexual matters; hypersexual by self-report 4 overt sexual acts (toward subjects, staff, or interviewer)
4. Sleep	0 reports no decrease in sleep 1 sleeping less than normal amount by up to one hour 2 sleeping less than normal by more than one hour 3 reports decreased need for sleep 4 denies need for sleep

5. Irritability	0	absent
	2	subjectively increased
	4	irritable at times during interview; recent episodes of anger or annoyance on ward
	6	frequently irritable during interview; short, curt throughout
	8	hostile, uncooperative; interview impossible
6. Speech (rate and amount)	0	no increase
	2	feels talkative
	4	increased rate or amount at times, verbose at times
	6	push; consistently increased rate and amount; difficult to interpret
	8	pressured; uninterruptible; continuous speech
7. Language-thought disorder	0	absent
	1	circumstantial; mild distractibility; quick thoughts
	2	distractible; loses goal of thought; changes topics frequently; racing thoughts
	3	flight of ideas; tangentiality; difficult to follow; rhyming; echolalia
	4	incoherent; communication impossible
8. Content	0	normal
	2	questionable plans, new interests
	4	special project(s); hyperreligious
	6	grandiose or paranoid ideas; ideas of reference
	8	delusions; hallucinations
9. Disruptive-aggressive behavior	0	absent, cooperative
	2	sarcastic; loud at times, guarded
	4	demanding; threats on ward
	6	threatens interviewer shouting; interview difficult
	8	assaultive; destructive; interview impossible
10. Appearance	0	appropriate dress and grooming
	1	minimally unkempt
	2	poorly groomed; moderately disheveled; overdressed
	3	disheveled; partly clothed; garish make-up
	4	completely unkempt; decorated; bizarre garb
11. Insight	0	present; admits illness; agrees with need fortreatment
	1	possibly ill
	2	admits behaviour change, but denies illness
	3	admits possible change in behaviour, but denies illness
	4	denies any behaviour change

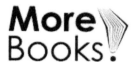
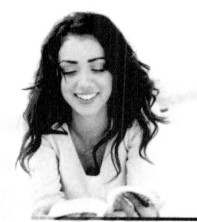
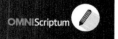

Printed in Great Britain
by Amazon

64358649R00058